Artificial Insemination of Small Ruminants

Artificial Insemination of Small Ruminants

R. Thiagarajan
Professor
Department of Animal Genetics and Breeding
Veterinary College and Research Institute
Tirunelveli-627 358

SATISH SERIAL PUBLISHING HOUSE
403, Express Tower, Commercial Complex
Azadpur, Delhi 110033 (India)
Phone : 011-27672852, Fax : 91-11-27672046
e-mail : info@satishserial.com, hkjain1975@yahoo.com
Website : www.satishserial.com

Published by :

SATISH SERIAL PUBLISHING HOUSE

403, Express Tower, Commercial Complex, Azadpur, Delhi-110033 (INDIA)
Phone : 011-27672852 Fax : 91-11-27672046
E-mail : info@satishserial.com, hkjain1975@yahoo.com

Reprint, 2019

ISBN 978-93-85055-62-1

Composed, Designed & Printed in India

Preface

The aim of writing this book is to provide an over-view about semen collection, semen evaluation, dilution, storage and freezing of semen and insemination in small ruminants. This book will be useful to under-graduate as well as post-graduate students of veterinary colleges in India.

I thank my wife Susila, daughter Kavya and son Thrishanth for their support, encouragement and patience during the preparation of this book.

I convey my sincere thanks to Satish Serial Publishing House, New Delhi for publishing this book.

R.Thiagarajan

Contents

PART-I :

ARTIFICIAL INSEMINATION IN GOATS

1

Introduction to Artificial Insemination in Goats

Perspectives in Goat Rearing

The Indian agriculture is traditionally characterized by mixed farming, combining field crop production with one or more of the livestock husbandry like raising of cattle, sheep, goat, pig and poultry. The prominent place of goat and sheep farming in the socio economic context of a landless and marginal but predominantly agrarian society can hardly be overstated. The National Commission on Agriculture recommend that as a method for providing additional rural employment and increasing milk and meat production in the country, livestock enterprises including dairy, goat and sheep husbandry be encouraged for the marginal, small and landless farmers.

Goats are the first among the domestic ruminants and considered as poor man's cow. Goats can be profitably raised with low investment under intensive and as well as the most extensive forms of nomadic grazing. Majority of the poor section of rural population depends on goat rearing for income and certain amount of meat and milk for home consumption. Goat rearing involves a low cost technology and therefore becomes handy to landless labourers, marginal farmers and industrial workers.

Goat population in India is 124.6 million (Livestock census, 2003), which is 15.32 % of the world's goat population. The population growth rate in India varied from 0.72 (1967-72) to 5.13% (1978-82) with an overall average of 3.5% during 1951-2003. In India, goats contribute to 22.27% of the milk, 10.86% of the meat and 13.3% of the fresh skins of the total productions of the world (FAO, 2004).

About 41% of goats of the total population are slaughtered every year for meat. The per capita annual availability of goat meat in the country is approximately 505 g and is 7.86% of the total meat and 3.0% of the total milk produced from all the species. Goats contribute to about Rs.10,087 crores, which is about 5.40% of the GNP contributed by the agriculture sector. The goat production systems are highly diversified in different parts of the country depending upon agro-ecological conditions and cropping systems. Therefore, development programmes in the country should be made region specific as per the requirement of region or sub-region.

With changes occurring rapidly in agriculture farming system due to mechanization, land use pattern, depletion of grazing land and high cropping intensity, the level of goat production, flock size, flock composition and goat population intensity is changing in different regions. The ultimate objective of goat production is to maximize profit from the available resources and production conditions in such a way suitable for socio-economic conditions of the poor farmers in different regions.

Limited access to good quality breeding bucks is one of the reasons for low productivity of goats. Artificial insemination, which has been standardized, could be used effectively as a breeding method for multiplication of superior quality animals. Studies have been conducted on sexual maturity and optimal age for semen production in different goat breeds. The deep cervical insemination technique with freshly diluted semen has been standardized with 75% fertility in goats. A fertility rate of 50% has been obtained with frozen semen using deep cervical insemination.

Artificial Insemination

Artificial insemination (AI) is a method of breeding in which semen is obtained from the male and introduced into the female reproductive tract by means of instruments.

Although AI has gained widespread acceptance in the dairy cattle industries of most developed countries, it has not yet received such universal acceptance in the sheep and goat breeding industries. There are several reasons for this. Often the cost of implementing an AI program has outweighed the economic benefit in an industry which sometimes operates on small profit margins; the cost and maintenance of breeding males can be relatively low; and the low success rate obtained in the past with the use of frozen semen in sheep and goats has been a limiting factor. However, recent technological advances have improved the efficiency of AI in sheep and goats.

Advantages of artificial insemination

1. Increased rate of genetic gain

The use of superior sires may have a direct effect on the production traits of the resultant progeny, and this may be all that the commercial producer requires. There will also be a long-term effect on production traits of future generations if the breeding program is continued. It naturally follows that genetic progress would be hastened by more widespread use of superior sires (selected on the basis of accurate estimates of breeding value), provided that problems of inbreeding do not arise.

The use of AI can greatly increase the number of offspring produced per sire per year. Using conventional flock/herd mating, a sire may be expected to mate 50-100 females per year. When fresh diluted semen is used with cervical insemination, a single buck could be used to inseminate in excess of 1000 females in a 2-3 week period. With intrauterine insemination of frozen-stored semen, many thousand does can be inseminated with semen collected from a single sire each year.

2. Easy transport of genetic material

Semen is much cheaper to transport than whole animals and is not subject to the same risks of spreading disease. AI has enabled new genes to be imported from overseas into countries, which will not allow importation of live animals. Thus, AI has made possible international exchange of semen.

3. Long-term-storage of semen

Semen from valuable males may be stored for use in future years, even after death, Many producers store semen from valuable males as insurance against their premature death, as well as to maximize their use in the shorter term.

4. Increased efficiency of breeding

Sub-fertile bucks may be readily identified and eliminated from the team of breeding males. Artificial insemination can also ensure that all females are mated, avoiding problems associated with male-female preferences, which often result in some oestrous females being missed at joining. If timed inseminations are used, females can be mated even if they do not display behavioural oestrus.

5. Reduction or elimination of the need to maintain males on farm

Small producers need not maintain any males on their own properties, provided they can obtain semen from outside sources. The cost and inconvenience of maintaining a team of breeding males can therefore be eliminated.

6. Prevention and control of disease

AI eliminates direct male-female contact and hence controls or prevents the spread of venereal and other diseases. It should be noted that AI is a prophylactic measure but is not a cure for disease.

7. Use of incapacitated males

Sometimes a particularly valuable male may have suffered injury or become infirm with age, preventing him from mating females. Provided that the semen of such a male is of sufficient quality, AI can enable his continued use for breeding.

8. Accurate record keeping

Use of AI permits accurate breeding records to be kept. Such records may be used to increase the accuracy of selection or to eliminate undesirable traits from the flock or herd.

9. Use in synchronized or out-of-season breeding

Producers may wish to make use of technology, which permits synchronized breeding of females. When practiced in large flocks or herds, synchronized breeding requires the use of AI, since it is not practicable to keep a sufficient number of males for natural mating. Out of season breeding programs may coincide with the time of year when semen quality is low; this is a problem in goats particularly. In this case it may be necessary to inseminate females with semen frozen and stored during the breeding season when semen quality is high.

10. Use of other technology

When females are superovulated for production of a large number of embryos for transfer, natural mating does not result in a high level of fertilization, Intrauterine insemination improves the fertilization rate and renders the technique viable. In addition, there has been some interest in pre-determining the sex of offspring. This could be achieved by separating the X and Y chromosome-bearing spermatozoa. If this technique is proved to be effective it will require AI with the segregated spermatozoa.

Disadvantages of artificial insemination

1. Inbreeding

When selection intensity is high, problems associated with inbreeding may arise. The extensive nature of the goat industries ensures that a large gene pool is maintained and inbreeding is unlikely to become a major problem. Nevertheless, care should be taken when using AI in a small, closed flock or herd.

2. Spread of disease

If the sire has not been properly tested for venereal disease, AI may spread the disease more rapidly than natural mating.

3. Reduced fertility

In comparison with natural insemination, AI may, under certain circumstances, result in reduced fertility, particularly when methods of controlling oestrus are not properly employed or the operator is careless or negligent when handling the semen.

4. Cost

As with any technology, production costs are incurred when AI is used. Such costs include the employment of skilled labour, equipment, drugs and hormones, recording, and purchase of semen or selection and maintenance of sires. As insemination equipment is simple and durable, equipment costs per insemination are relatively low. Since fewer males are required for AI than for natural mating, total sire costs can be reduced.

❑❑❑

2

Anatomy of the Female Reproductive Tract

The basic organs of a doe are the ovaries, oviducts, uterus, cervix, and vagina. With regard to artificial insemination, the most important difference between the two ewe and doe is in the cervix.

The ovaries

The ovaries are the female gonads or primary sex organs, and correspond to the testes of the male. Each female has two ovaries, which are usually equally active. They have two basic functions, (i) production of female gametes called ova. (or eggs), and (ii) production of the female sex hormones, predominantly progesterone and oestrogen, which are essential for the development and maintenance of female characteristics, rcproduction, and lactation.

The ovaries are located in the abdominal cavity behind the kidneys, and are supported by the broad utero-ovarian ligament. This maintains them in close proximity to the uterine horns.

The surface of each ovary is covered by a single layer of flattened cells known as the germinal epithelium. Underneath is a layer tough, dense connective tissue, the tunica albuginea, which surrounds the cortex, or enter region of the ovary. The cortex is made up of ovarian stroma, follicles at various stages of development, and corpora lutea or corpora albicantia. The ovaries are well supplied with blood vessels.

Each ovarian follicle contains a single oocyte, which develops into a ripe (fertilizable) ovum. A large follicle has an antrum, a fluid-filled cavity surrounded by the follicle wall. The theca and granulose cells are responsible for follicular hormone production, predominantly oestrogen. After release of the ovum at ovulation, the follicle becomes transformed into a solid yellow body 0.5-1.0 cm in diameter, the corpus luteum, which secretes progesterone. At the end of the oestrous cycle, the corpus luteum becomes pale in colour and transforms into an inactive corpus albicans, resembling scar tissue, and gradually disappears.

The Oviducts

The two oviducts (or fallopian tubes) thin, tortuous tubes, each 10-20 cm long, extending from the ovaries to the uterine horns. They are supported by a thin membrane (the mesosalpinx), which is part of the broad ligament supporting the uterus. The function of the oviducts is to pick up eggs from the ovaries and transport them to the uterus, and to act as the site of fertilization.

The ovarian end of each oviduct opens into a wide funnel like process called the, infundibulum. Passage of the ovum to the infundibulum is facilitated by the sticky mass of cumulus oophorus cells which surround the ovum at ovulation, but which are lost within a matter of hours thereafter. Despite the open nature of the infundibulum, few ova are lost into the abdominal cavity. Further transport along the tubes is achieved by the beating of cilia lining the inner surface of the oviducts.

The infundibulum leads to the initial segment of the oviduct, a relatively broad tubal portion called the ampulla. It is here spermatozoa swimming up the tube encounter the ovum and fertilization occurs. The fertilized ovum, or zygote or embryo as it is now called, then travels down the remaining portion of the tube, which is a relatively narrow section called the isthmus. The oviducts join the uterus at the utero-tubal junction.

There are glandular cells in the wall of the oviduct; these secrete fluids, which maintain the ovum or embryo. Although the embryo does not grow considerably during its time in the oviduct, it requires a finely balanced nutrient medium to ensure normal development. If passage of the embryo into the uterus occurs prematurely, then the embryo will die.

The Uterus

This organ consists of two horns and a body. In does the two uterine horns (9-16 cm long) are joined at the bifurcation. The body of the uterus is short (3-5 cm), and is divided close to the bifurcation by a short septum, which does not extend all the way to the cervix and allows passage of pre implementation embryos from one horn to the other. Implantation of an embryo and development as a foetus occurs within one of the horns of the uterus. A single ovulation will result in implantation of the embryo in the adjacent uterine horn; multiple embryos originating from the same ovary tend to distribute themselves equally between the two horns.

The endometrium is a glandular layer, which hypertrophies under the influence of progesterone and secretes nutrients for the embryo before implantation. Foetal attachment occurs at special sites called caruncles; there is 70-100 of these mushroom-like projections lining the interior surface of the horns.

The Cervix

The cervix is 4-7 cm long and connects the uterus to the anterior vagina. It has a relatively hard structure comprising connective tissue, musculature, and secretory glands on the inner ling. These glands produce cervical mucus and are particularly active at oestrus. The spermatozoa must swim through the cervical mucus to reach the uterus.

The internal wall of the cervix has a number of ridges and crypts, which fit together so as to, make the cervix directly impassable. This has the effect of sealing on the uterus from the vagina, thereby keeping out infection. In goat does, however, the lumen is much more open, particularly at oestrus, and an inseminating pipette can be inserted well into the cervix, and through it in 30-50% of animals.

The Vagina

The vagina is the female organ in which semen is deposited during copulation in goats. It can also be regarded as a common passage for both the urinary and reproductive systems.

The anterior part of the vagina, which contains the entrance to the cervix, forms a recess, called the vaginal fornix. During natural mating semen is deposited in this part of the vagina. Posterior to the vaginal fornix is the vestibule, a short, narrower portion that closes the vagina off from the exterior. The urethral orifice is located in the lower posterior part of the vestibule. The vestibule also contains secretory glands, which produce mucus to lubricate the vagina when the female is in oestrus.

During oestrus it is moist and has a red flush. Females with a dry, pale-looking vagina are probably not in oestrus and there would be little chance of conception after insemination at this time.

The external and terminal part of the vagina is the vulva. In the doe it has a triangular form, with the tip down. The vulva may also have a red flush at oestrus.

❑❑❑

3

Physiology of Reproduction in Does

Maturation of Ovarian Follicles and Ova

The ovaries of the female at birth contain all the ova necessary for her reproductive life, and no more new, ova are produced after birth. Although only a few dozen ova may ever be ovulated, the ovaries contain several hundred thousand ova. Many of these degenerate, particularly during the early life of the animal, but others grow and mature into fertile ova after puberty.

The small ova, called oogonia, in the ovaries of female foetuses are diploid cells. They multiply by mitotic division before birth. After birth they undergo a period of growth and then enter the first meiotic division, at which point development is temporarily arrested. They are known as primary oocytes at is stage. Each primary oocyte is surrounded by a layer of flattened cells, and together they form a primary follicle.

The primary follicle remains inactive until sexual maturity of the female, at which time some of them begin to grow. The oocyte enlarges and acquires a jelly-like transparent outer layer, or shell, the zona pellucida. The primary follicle increases in size to become a secondary follicle and, subsequently, a tertiary follicle with an antrum. As the follicle further matures, to become a Graafian follicle, it appears as a blister-like structure, up to 1 cm in diameter, on the surface of the ovary. During the final maturation of the follicle the first meiotic division is completed and the first polar body (containing surplus chromosomes) is extended. The oocyte is now known as a secondary oocyte, and it, is this stage that the follicle ruptures and releases the ovum: the process called ovulation. The second meiotic division, completed only when the ovum is activated after penetration by a fertilizing spermatozoon, and the second polar body is extruded.

The Oestrous Cycle

Goat does exhibit oestrus, or heat, at regular intervals during the breeding season. Oestrus is the fertile period and if the female does not conceive, it is repeated every 19-21 days in goat does (normal range 17-24 days). The repeating chain of events leading to regular oestrous periods is called the oestrous cycle.

For simplicity, the oestrous cycle may be divided into two phases, the follicular phase (the period of follicular growth) and the luteal phase (the period of the corpus luteum). Oestrus occurs during the later stages, of the follicular phase. The follicular phase is relatively short, only 3-4 days in goat does, and the luteal phase occupies the rest of the cycle (about 17 days in does).

Follicular Phase

Follicular growth is under the control of the two gonadotrophins released by the pituitary gland, namely follicle stimulating hormones (FSH) and luteinising hormone (LH). FSH stimulates the early growth of the follicles and, in addition, LH is necessary to complete the later growth phases. As well as promoting follicular growth, the gonadotrophins stimulate the growing follicle to secrete the female sex hormone oestrogen, which is released into the bloodstream. Graafian follicles produce relatively large amounts of oestrogen. At first, the relatively low level of oestrogen in the blood feeds back to the pituitary gland and has a negative (inhibitory) effect on gonadotrophin secretion. This helps to prevent excessive stimulation of the ovaries. However, when the level of oestrogen in the blood is high enough it triggers the release of a surge of LH from the pituitary gland. This so called preovulatory LH surge brings about changes in the wall of the follicle, causing it to rupture and release the ovum. The LH surge also triggers the meiotic maturation of the oocyte (conversion of a primary oocyte to a secondary oocyte).

The oestrogen circulating in the bloodstream during the follicular phase is primarily responsible for induction of oestrous behaviour in females. The level of oestrogen in the blood rises and reaches a peak just before the onset of oestrus. The preovulatory LH surge occurs early in oestrus and is followed by ovulation some 18-24 hours later.

Apart from oestrogen the maturing follicle also produces the hormone inhibin, which selectively inhibits secretion of FSH by the pituitary gland. By limiting FSH secretion, inhibin prevents the growth of additional follicles in the presence of Graafian follicles and thereby helps to limit ovulation rate.

Luteal Phase

After ovulation, the ruptured Graafian follicle is filled with a blood clot and becomes a red body known as a corpus haemorrhagicum. Under the influence of the LH surge, the granulose cells in the wall reptured follicle proliferate and transform into lutin cells, which subsequently fill the antrum of the follicle. Over 4-5 days the corpus haemorrhagicum is transformed into a solid yellow body, the corpus luteum. The whole process is known as luteinisation.

The corpus luteum secretes the female sex hormone, progesterone. Progesterone prepares the uterus for acceptance of a fertilized ovum or embryo. The progesterone level in the blood stream reaches a peak after about 6 days, and remains high throughout pregnancy if the animal conceives. If the animal fails to conceive, after 13-14 days in the goat doe, the corpus luteum decreases in size, becomes pale in colour (a corpus albicans) and its progesterone secretion begins to fall. Since a high blood progesterone level has an inhibitory influence on secretion of gonadotrophins by the pituitary gland, follicular growth is limited. Removal of the inhibition at the end of the luteal phase leads to a new wave of follicular growth, and the cycle progresses.

The demise of the corpus luteum is brought about by a luteolytic agent, prostaglandin-F2α, which is produced by the uterus after prolonged progesterone stimulation. If the animal becomes pregnant, prostaglandin-F2α, production is suppressed and the corpus luteum remains active. Synthetic prostaglandins have been used to destroy the corpus luteum prematurely during the oestrous cycle. Such treatment, which is followed by a new wave of follicular growth, can be used to synchronize oestrus and ovulation.

Oestrus

Oestrus (or heat) is the period of the oestrous cycle when the female displays behavioural sexual activity, and it is the only time that she will accept the male. Oestrus occurs during the mid to late-follicular phase of the cycle. Oestrogen secreted by large follicles is responsible for the anatomical and behavioural changes associated with oestrus.

The signs of oestrus are much more marked in the goat doe. The outward signs include reddening of the vulva and vaginal discharge of mucus; accompanied by restless behaviour, tail wagging and nuzzling or nudging of the male. Goat does in oestrus display homosexual behaviour that is a doe in oestrus may mount other females in the herd. In goat herds teaser males may be used to detect oestrous females. The only sure sign of oestrus is if the female will stand and allow the male to mount (the 'standing reflex'). The male detects a female in oestrus by the characteristic odour of the vaginal secretion.

Although the male is usually considered to be the aggressive partner, a female in oestrus will often see out the male and force her attentions upon him. Thus, a male can often be seen with a 'harem' of oestrous females surrounding him, competing for his attention. This allows for male preference in choosing mates and, as a result some females in oestrus may not be mated or marked by a teaser male. Young females, which do not show aggressive oestrous behaviour, may be overlooked in a mixed flock or herd containing mature females.

During oestrus there are increases in the blood flow and in the secretory activity of the glands of the uterus, cervix and vagina. The vulva and vagina may become congested. There is abundant secretion of mucus, which collects in the vagina or, occasionally, flows from the vulva. This type and consistency of the mucus changes through the oestrus period, and this can be used to estimate the stage of oestrus in relation to the appropriate time for insemination. At the beginning of oestrus the mucus is clear and sparse, after 12-18 hours it is clear to cloudy and copious, and at 25-30 hours becomes thicker and creamier in consistency.

The duration of oestrus in does varies from 16 to 50 hours. This period varies with breed, age, geographical location and contact with males. Oestrus is shorter in young females than in mature ones. Oestrus is also shorter if females are continually exposed to males than if they have intermittent contact or are 'hand teased'. In mature does, the duration of oestrus is usually 20-40 hours, and 18-30 hours in young does. It has been shown that females with short oestrous periods (under 24 hours) are less fertile than those with longer oestrous periods. This may be related to the number of ovulations, since animals with short oestrous periods rarely have twin ovulations. However, there appears to be no relationship between the duration of oestrus and the number of ovulation in females with oestrus of 24-60 hours duration.

Ovulation

Ovulation is the process in which the mature Graafian follicle ruptures and releases the ripe ovum. In does, ovulation is spontaneous, that is, it occurs regardless of whether or not mating takes place.

Time of Ovulation

The time of ovulation is related to the onset of oestrus; in goat does about 30-36 hours after the onset of oestrus. Thus, ovulation generally occurs late in oestrus, though in females with short oestrous periods it may occur after the end of oestrus. When two or more follicle mature in the same oestrous cycle the ova are usually related within 2-3 hours of each other.

Accurate knowledge of the time of ovulation is crucial to the success of insemination since the ovulated ova have only a short fertilizable life, insemination should be carried out so that the spermatozoa reach the oviducts close to the time of ovulation. Later insemination may result in reduced fertility.

Ovulation Rate

Ovulation rate (number of eggs released at ovulation) is determined by the number of follicles, which develop to the Graafian stage. The ovulation rate partly determines the number of offspring that a female will carry. Multiple ovulation also improves the chances of conception. In general, goats have higher ovulation rates, but there are a number of factors, which influence the ovulation rate of each species. These include genetic factors, live weight, nutritional status and age of the animal, and season: Some breed of goats have higher ovulation rates than others.

Ovulation rate increases with age and reaches a peak at 3-5 years. In most females the ovulation rate increases from the beginning of the breeding season to a maximum in mid-season, and then declines as anoestrus approaches.

Breeding Season

Goats display marked changes in breeding activity from season to season. They are called short day breeders since their breeding season begins when days are shortening, that is in the autumn.

The length of the breeding season varies with species, breed, nutrition and lactation status of the animal. Animals in poor condition may have a short breeding season, or may fail to show oestrus altogether.

In anoestrus, the pituitary gland is relatively inactive and secretes very little gonadotrophin into the bloodstream. Consequently, follicular growth is not stimulated, and the female does not display oestrus or ovulate. At the beginning of the breeding season, pituitary activity increases the gonadotrophin levels raise and stimulate growth and maturation of the follicles.

Ovarian activity increases gradually as a new breeding season approaches. Thus, there is a transitory period between the non breeding and breeding seasons when gonadotrophin levels gradually begin to rise in the bloodstream, but not sufficiently so to cause oestrus and ovulation. Nevertheless, females at this stage are highly responsive to artificial stimulation of ovulation, such as by injection of gonadotrophins. Introduction of a buck to isolated females (the buck effect) is also effective in stimulating ovulation during the transitory period, and the response is more marked in goats.

Through stimulation of oestrus and ovulation before the normal onset of the breeding season, producers may have offspring ready for early markets when prices are relatively high. Producers may also wish to stimulate breeding activity at the middle of anoestrus, for example so that lambing may coincide with favourable climatic conditions or to ensure year round milk production in the case of dairy goats. Controlled breeding techniques used in conjunction with artificial insemination can permit year-round breeding in most breeds. Breeds, which have short breeding seasons may be more difficult to breed out of season since they apparently, have a greater depth of anoestrus than other breeds.

Transport of Spermatozoa in the Female Reproductive Tract

During artificial insemination, the semen may be deposited into the entrance to the cervix or, in some cases, into the anterior cervix or uterus. When semen is deposited in this manner, successful insemination can be achieved with fewer spermatozoa than when semen is deposited into the vagina.

Survival of spermatozoa is generally thought to be better in the cervix than in other regions of the female tract. After semen deposition in the vagina or cervix, a 'sperm reservoir' becomes established in the folds and crypts of the cervix. The reservoir supplies spermatozoa to the uterus and oviducts over a considerable period (24 hours or more). There is also evidence to suggest that a second sperm reservoir is formed in the utero tubal junction and/or isthmus region of oviduct. Maximum numbers of spermatozoa can be found in the oviducts 12-24 hours after insemination. The establishment of a sperm reservoir in the cervix is not necessary after intrauterine insemination (either by laparoscopy, or through the cervix in some goats).

The swimming action of spermatozoa maintains them in suspension in the cervical and uterine fluids. Spermatozoa move through the female tract sweep the uterine fluids containing suspended spermatozoa towards the oviducts. The uterine contractions are stimulated by oestrogen secreted by the ovarian follicles. Restraint of does at insemination may cause stress, which could be a factor interfering with uterine contractions and therefore with transport of spermatozoa to the oviducts.

Fertilization

Fertilization is the fusion of an ovum and a spermatozoon, which results in the formation of a diploid cell. The new diploid cell (with 2n chromosomes) is called an embryo or zygote.

The site of fertilization is the ampulla, a broad region of the oviduct. For fertilization to occur, there must be no obstacle for the spermatozoa and the ova to meet in the oviduct (one of both oviducts may be blocked in a small proportion of females). After ovulation, the ovum is swept down the oviduct to the ampulla by the beating action of cilia on the inner lining of the infundibulum and the oviduct wall. When spermatozoa meet the ovum, the head of one spermatozoon penetrates the zona pellucida surrounding the ovum. Penetration is aided by enzymes released from the acrosome of the sperm cell, which digest an opening through the zona pellucida, and by whiplash motion of the sperm tail. Although only a single spermatozoon fuses with the ovum, many more spermatozoa are required in the uterus and oviducts to ensure that fertilization occurs.

Spermatozoa survive in the uterus and oviducts for only 10-12 hours. The life of the ovulated ovum is 12-24 hours. If either the spermatozoon or the ovum is aged, then penetration of the ovum may not occur or, if it does, the resultant embryo may develop abnormally and degenerate. It is therefore important that insemination occurs close to ovulation.

❑❑❑

4

Preparation of Females for Insemination and Synchronization of Oestrus

Several weeks before the start of an AI program attention should be paid to the condition of the females and their preparation for insemination. The success of the program is dependent on the fertility of the females as much as on the quality of semen used for insemination.

Artificial insemination is successful only if performed at a fixed time in relation to ovulation, or to the onset of oestrus. It is therefore necessary to either (i) detect oestrus in females which are cycling naturally, or (ii) control, or synchronize, Oestrus synchronization may be associated with reduced fertility, and they can also be costly in terms of materials or labour; there may therefore be some advantage in using the natural oestrus detection method. However, synchronization of oestrus has the advantage of shortening the time taken to inseminate a whole flock or herd, and it facilitates management during pregnancy and parturition. In addition, control of oestrus makes it possible to stimulate ovulation artificially, there by increasing fertility (number of females conceiving) and fecundity (number of offspring per female). When exogenous gonadotrophins are used to stimulate ovulation there is the added advantage that the time over which ovulation occurs is decreased, that is, the treatment increases the synchrony of ovulation and hence the success of fixed time inseminations. Stimulation of oestrus and ovulation may also be effective in the non-breeding season, permitting out of season breeding.

Condition of Females for Insemination

As for natural mating, females to be included in an AI program should be in good health, free of diseases and parasites, and in good body condition. Sick or malnourished females will often fail to ovulate or suffer a high rate of embryo mortality. In general, heavier females have a higher ovulation rate than lighter females in the same flock or herd. They should not be over-fat, as this may result in reproductive disorders. Lambs or kids should be weaned at least 6-8 weeks before insemination of their dams. Stressful procedures should be avoided for 6-8 weeks before and 4 weeks after insemination. These procedures include all sanitary or prophylactic measures such as dipping, drenching, vaccination, shearing and crutching.

Identification of Females

To enable accurate records to be kept, each female should be clearly identifiable. If individual breeding records are to be kept each female should have a numbered ear tag. Groups of females may be tagged with coloured tags, each colour corresponding to an individual sire, to facilitate sorting at a later time. To avoid stress or inconvenience at the time of insemination, it is best if ear tags are put in place before hand, for example at the time of selection of females to enter the AI program, at drafting of oestrous females, or at the time of progestogen or prostaglandin treatment. However, if ear tagging is done before insemination, ear tags must be removed from any females, which are not inseminated for any reason. Any of the commercial ear tags are suitable, but to avoid delays at the time of insemination it is best if the ear tag numbers are prominent enough to be quickly identified.

Time of year for Insemination

Goat does are generally joined or inseminated during the natural breeding season. When oestrus and ovulation are induced, however does can be inseminated at any time of the year, providing semen of sufficient quality is available. It may be possible to obtain fresh semen of good quality in the non-breeding season only from the less seasonal breeds of goats; it is virtually impossible in some breeds. Instead, good quality semen can be collected in the breeding season and frozen stored for later use.

Best insemination results are usually obtained in the natural breeding season, particularly in goats. Nevertheless, local pasture growth or market forces may make it worthwhile to breed outside the normal season.

Drafting of Females in Natural Oestrus

Insemination of females in natural oestrus is restricted to the breeding season. As we have seen, the length of the oestrous cycle is about 21 days in goat does. Since the oestrous period lasts for about 24-42 hours, then we can expect that 5-7% of does will be on heat each day of the breeding season. It also follows that it takes atleast 21 days to inseminate a herd of does.

The females in oestrus must be identified and drafted off from the main flock or herd. Even though goat does exhibit visible signs of oestrus more clearly than ewes teaser bucks should be employed for reliable heat detection.

To avoid the potential problem of reduced fertility due to a synchronization treatment, a combination of the methods of synchronization of oestrus (1st cycle) and detection of oestrous females at the subsequent (2nd cycle) oestrus can be used. This results in most females coming in (natural) oestrus over a period of 4-5 days. However, there is usually little merit in the use of combined treatments as synchronization treatment alone, when used correctly, results in acceptable fertility levels and is much more convenient.

Synchronization of Oestrus

There are several methods of synchronization of oestrus. They fall into two major categories, namely the pharmacological or natural methods. The pharmacological methods are effective in closely synchronizing oestrus in the majority of females in flock or herd, and predetermined fixed-time insemination can be practiced, but they do incur some expense in the purchase and administration of the pharmacological produces. The natural method may be less expensive, but does not result in close synchronization of oestrus.

Pharmacological Methods of Oestrus Synchronization

The pharmacological methods can be divided into two types, based on different physiological principles. The first type is based on administration of synthetic progestogens (or progesterone) to simulate the action of a natural corpus luteum. The second type is based on administration of prostaglandin -F2α or synthetic prostaglandins to shorten the life of corpora lutea. Since the prostaglandin method depends on the presence of a corpus luteum, it can only be used in the breeding season. The progestogen method can be used at any time of the year.

1. Progestogen method

When progestogen is administered daily for 16-18 days in does, oestrus and ovulation do not occur. On termination of this treatment, oestrus usually occurs 2-3 days later. The treatment acts in the same way as a corpus luteum, and pituitary output of gonadotrophins is suppressed. Once the progestogen treatment is withdrawn, the pituitary releases increasing amounts of gonadotrophins, which stimulate the growth, and subsequent ovulation of follicles. Exogenous progestogen treatment does not affect the function of a fully formed corpus luteum. For effective synchronization of a group of females, therefore, the duration of progestogen treatment must equal or exceed the lifespan of a corpus luteum (16-18 days in goats).

There are several methods of administrating progestogens (or progesterone) to goat does. The most convenient methods involve handling the females twice only, once to insert a progestogen-releasing device, and once to remove it. At removal, ovulation-stimulating treatments can also be administered.

Both the intravaginal and the subcutaneous routes have been used for administration of exogenous progestogens. For convenience and simplicity, intravaginal devices are preferable. They are of two forms, the intravaginal pessary or sponges, and the CIDR (Controlled Internal Drug Release dispenser). The CIDR has not been tested under sufficiently varied conditions to determine accurately its effects on fertility. Subcutaneous implants are also manufactured but are not available in some areas.

a) The progestogen pessary or sponge

These devices are manufactured under the names of Chronogest® (Intervet) or lepromap® (Upjohn). Chronogest® sponges contain 30, 40 or 45 mg fluorogestone acetate (FGA) as synthetic progestogen. Sponges containing 45 mg for goat does are recommended at all times. The 40 mg sponges are suitable for maiden animals. Repromap® sponges contain 60 mg of medroxyprogesterone acetate (MAP), and are-used-for-all-purposes. Essentially there is no difference in effectiveness of the two brands of sponges, though experimental reports have occasionally favoured one type over the other.

Each intravaginal sponge is threaded with a string to aid withdrawal. The sponge is inserted into the vagina with the aid of an applicator, which consists of a plastic tube and rod.

Insertion of sponges: Insertion of sponges is done in a race capable of holding 20-30 females. Each sponge should be treated with an antibiotic powder or cream before insertion. The applicator should also be moistened with an antiseptic solution, which helps to lubricate as well as disinfect the applicator. The sponge is placed in the wide end or the tube and pushed to the front (beveled) end with the rod in such a manner that the string dangles through the tube and protrudes at the rear. The tube, with the rod placed inside, is then inserted gently into the vagina of the female to depth of 10-15 cm. This should not require much force. The female should be in a natural standing position; if she is in a twisted or kneeling position the vaginal wall may be perforated by the applicator. Once in position, the sponge is pushed from the tube with the rod, leaving it in the anterior vagina. On careful withdrawal of the applicator the string should protrude about 15-20 cm from the vagina. The applicator should be carefully disinfected (in a bucket containing antiseptic solution) between treatments of each female to avoid the spread of infection.

When a good race, handling cords and several applicators are available, a team of three men can treat up to 200 females per hour. It is the best when one member of the team disinfects and loads the sponges in to the applicators while the other two insert the sponges.

Maiden females may have tight vaginas. In this case it may wise to avoid using the applicator and push the sponge into the vagina with a finger instead. Special narrow sponges for maiden females are commercially available.

Removal of sponges: The sponges are removed after the recommended insertion period. As for sponge insertion, this can be done most conveniently in a race. The protruding string should be pulled outwards and lightly downwards, firmly but smoothly. Withdrawal is often accompanied by a discharge of distinctive smelling fluid from the vagina; this is normal, except when the discharge contains blood or pus signifying vaginal damage or infection. Such females should be treated with antibiotics and discarded from the insemination pool.

When sponges are properly inserted the loss rate is no more than- 1-2%; - Females without sponges will not come on heat at the appropriate time and should be reserved for insemination or mating at a later date. Occasionally, the string of the sponge creeps up into the vagina and out of sight. If a string cannot be seen protruding from the vulva it is best not to assume that the sponge has been lost; one should check for the presence of a sponge in the vagina. This can be done with the aid of a speculum, and the sponge, if present, removed with long forceps. This procedure will also be necessary on occasions when the string pulls through the sponge during attempted removal. Used sponges should be collected together and burned or buried.

After withdrawal of the sponges, the majority of females will come into heat within 2-3 days in the breeding season. Fertility of females inseminated at this first oestrus is usually lower than in untreated females, but this can be overcome by (i) double cervical insemination with a relatively high number of spermatozoa. (ii) intrauterine insemination, (iii) treatment with exogenous gonadotrophins to stimulate oestrus and ovulation, or (iv) introduction of 5-10% teaser males at the time of sponge withdrawal to stimulate oestrus and ovulation. These remedies may be used separately or in combination.

b) The subcutaneous implant

Oestrus can be controlled effectively using progestogen impregnated subcutaneous implants. They are put in place, usually under the skin of the ear or under the pit of the foreleg by means of a special applicator with a sharp needle. Removal is achieved by cutting the skin with a scalpel and withdrawing the implant with sterile forceps. This method is as effective as the intravaginal sponge, but it has not gained popularity as a means of controlling oestrus in goats since the surgical procedures involved are time consuming, somewhat stressful to the animal, and open wounds which may become infected.

If implants are to be used, the insertion period and treatments for enhancing fertility are similar to those used for intravaginal sponges.

2. Prostaglandin method

When does are in the mid to late luteal phase of the oestrous cycle, the corpus luteum can be destroyed by prostaglandin-F2". The inhibitory effect of progesterone, produced by the corpus luteum, on the pituitary gland is thereby removed and the pituitary releases increasing amount of gonadotrophins. The gonadotrophins stimulate follicular growth and oestrus occurs within 2-3 days.

Synthetic prostaglandins, such as Cloprostenol (Estrumate®, ICI) and Prosolvin (Intervet) are available in injectable form. These are more potent than the natural form. A dose of 125 mg of Cloprostenol is effective in causing luteal regression in sheep and goats. The manufacturer's recommended dose for Prosolvin® is 3.75 mg for goats. Lutalyse® (Upjohn) is a natural form of prostaglandin; 7.5 mg is reported to be an effective dose for goats. The manufacturer's recommended dose for Prosolvin® is 3.75 mg for goats. Prostaglandins are administered by intramuscular injection. It should be noted that the corpus luteum is only responsive to prostaglandins between days 6-17 in goats. For complete synchronization of the whole flock or herd, therefore, two injections are required, spaced 10-14 days apart in does; sire studies have shown a clear advantage for a 14 day injection interval over shorter intervals. Oestrus normally occurs in a high proportion of females within 2-3 days of the secondary injection.

There is wide variability in the response of goats to prostaglandins, and fertility at the induced oestrus is generally lower than after progestogen sponge treatment. To overcome the reduction in fertility, the same remedial measures as are used with the second prostaglandins injection. There are, however, other disadvantages of prostaglandins in oestrus control. They cannot be used in females, which are not cycling naturally, for example in the non-breeding season, and they are generally more expensive to use than the progestogen methods.

Natural Method of Oestrus Control (Male effect)

The natural method of oestrus induction or synchronization has been described variously as the male effect, teaser effect, or more specifically as the buck effect, teaser effect. In simple terms it involves introduction of males to females which have been previously isolated from males for several weeks. If the females are to be artificially inseminated the males should, of course, be sterile (teasers). This method of oestrus synchronization has proved to be effective only at certain times of the year, usually just before the onset of a natural breeding season, when the majority of females are not yet cycling. It is not effective when females are already cycling, nor in the deep anoestrous period of the more seasonal breeds of goats. The induced oestrus is not synchronized closely enough for times inseminations to be successful, and teaser males must be employed for accurate oestrus detection. However, the method has gained some favour due to its simplicity and relatively low cost, particularly in areas where sheep are routinely bred before the beginning of the natural breeding season.

If the male effect is to be employed, its use is recommended only in the period just before the normal breeding season. The females should be isolated from all contact with males, including, sight, smell and sound, for a period of at least 4 weeks. Teaser males, which may be fitted with harnesses and crayons, are introduced at a rate of at least 4%. Most does will exhibit fertile oestrus within 24 days and goat does within 30 days. In goat does, the first oestrus occurs at the beginning of the breeding season is not usually silent, and the buck effect result in a high level of synchronization of oestrus. However, in goat does too, short cycles of 5-6 or 10-12 days may occur after introduction of males, and the fertility is lower than for full cycles.

It should be noted that the male effect varies in its effectiveness with several factors, including location, time of year in relation to be breeding season, breed, nutritional status and age of the animals. It is advisable to test the method under local conditions before implementing a large AI program based on the technique.

Stimulation of Ovulation

Most breeds of goats are capable of carrying and rearing litters of at least two offspring. This represents a source of potential reproductive wastage, and can be remedied by stimulation of the ovulation rate of females at oestrus. Also, it is usually necessary to stimulate ovulation when goats are to be inseminated outside their regular breeding season.

Ideally, to achieve an average of two offspring one should aim to stimulation ovulation rate of about three ova, as there will be subsequent losses through fertilization failure and embryo mortality. The methods used to stimulate ovulation in AI programs usually have the added advantages of stimulating oestrous behaviour, improving the synchrony of ovulation, and improving overall fertility. Care should be taken to use only mild stimulation, thereby avoiding an excessively high degree of superovulation.

Ovulation rate can be stimulated by either pharmacological or natural methods. Some pharmacological methods require that oestrus be synchronized, whereas the natural methods can be used alone or in conjunction with oestrus synchronization.

Pharmacological Methods of Stimulation of Ovulation

These methods are based on supplementation of the natural pituitary gonadotrophins (FSH and LH) with exogenous gonadotrophins in the follicular phase of the oestrous cycle. This helps to stimulate growth of one or more extra follicles to the point of ovulation, and thereby the release of more ova for fertilization.

Supplementation of Gonadotrophin

The exogenous gonadotrophins most commonly used for stimulation of ovulation are either extracts of the pituitaries of horses or pigs, or of the serum of pregnant mares. The pituitary extracts are short-acting and require frequent injection to sustain the stimulation and, though they have value when a high degree of superovulation is required, their use is inconvenient in large AI programmes. Pregnant mare serum gonadotrophin (PMSG) is more commonly used since it is relatively long acting and required only a single injection.

PMSG can be injected either intramuscularly or subcutaneously in 1-2 ml of sterile saline or water (usually supplied with the freeze-dried PMSG). Dissolve the PMSG in the saline or water just before use. It is best to inject into the fleshy or muscular part of the hind leg or rump, or under the skin of the pit of the leg. The does to be used depends on the breed of animal and the season. Large animals of breeds of relatively poor fertility will require higher doses, as well animals in the non-breeding season. As a general rule the doses of PMSG should be 400-500 IU for females in the natural breeding season and 600-750 IU for those in the non-breeding season.

It is necessary to synchronize oestrus before injection of PMSG. The PMSG may be injected at any time during the 2 days before the time withdrawal of the progestogen treatment (pessary or implant) or injection of prostaglandin. In practice, it is convenient to inject PMSG at the same time as removal of the pessary/implants or injection of prostaglandin. It has been noted, however, that injection of PMSG 1-2 days before withdrawal of the progestogen treatment may be more effective in the non-breeding season, particularly in goats.

PMSG is a natural product and varies considerably in its chemical composition, and sometimes in its biological action. Although the manufacturing companies make every effort to standardize each batch, some batch variation has been experienced from time to time. This may occasionally result in an ovulation rate higher or lower than expected, especially when coupled with individual animal or group variation in response to PMSG. PMSG should therefore be purchased from a reputable source and used with caution.

Recommended method for controlled breeding in does

DAY	GOAT	
	Breeding season	**Non-breeding season**
0	Insert Sponges 45 mg FGA or 60 mg MAP	
14		Inject PMSG 600-750 IU
16	Remove Sponge Inject PMSG 400 I.U	
	Introduce 5-10% teaser males*	
18	Inseminate	

(*) The requirement for teaser bucks has not been fully evaluated and this is a suggested number only.

Note: Responses of the animals to PMSG may vary depending on breed, nutrition, stage of breeding season etc. as incorrect use of PMSG can have adverse effects, it would be wise to consult local experts with regard to the correct dose to be used before undertaking a large program.

□□□

5

Handling of Frozen Semen

The quality of frozen semen plays an imported role in deciding the conception rate in bovines especially in the field. The quality is affected due to mishandling of frozen straws during transfer, storage and during insemination. There is also a possibility of transmission of pathogenic bacteria and viruses through semen. Lack of appropriate measures during handling and maintenance of frozen semen may lower the quality of semen and subsequent conception. Semen therefore should be properly handled and maintained once it has reached the insemination center. There are chances of deteriorating good quality semen without our knowledge due to many lapses while handling and using it. The frozen semen collected at the semen production stations is handled at different places before being used for insemination. Strict quality control measures are to be exercised at all levels for obtaining maximum results. The quality of the semen being distributed to the AI centers has to be ensured. Maintenance of cold chain of semen in liquid nitrogen will also have to be assured.

The spermatozoa are affected by cryoinjury during freezing and thawing. The thawed spermatozoa are very fragile and if exposed again to thermal shock during our handling results in poor fertility. Sufficient care should be taken during transfer of semen straws from storage container to field containers, during thawing, during loading of the insemination gun and while insemination. While handling of frozen semen the influence of fluctuation of temperature should be minimized. There should not be any contamination with pathogenic bacteria and the temperature shock should be avoided.

Thawing and insemination are the two important phases to be handled by the inseminator with utmost care. Theoretically faster a sperm is frozen, the more rapidly it should be thawed for optimal survival. The most widely practiced temperature range 37^{0}C for 30 seconds is suitable to get optimum survival of spermatozoa.

Storage of frozen semen

1. The frozen semen straws must always be kept submerged in liquid nitrogen.
2. Frozen semen containers should be periodically topped with liquid nitrogen.
3. Straws must be stored in a plastic goblet, which in turn is fitted into a canister.
4. Always keep identification slip or coloured plastic sticks in the goblet to enable quick identification.

The goblets must be slightly shorter than straws to enable quick removal of straws. Frozen semen should never be touched with fingers. Long stainless steel forceps may be used for handling the frozen straws. To avoid any raise in temperature, the forceps or any object, which is to come in contact with frozen semen, should be immersed in liquid nitrogen before the frozen straw is handled.

Thawing of frozen semen

1. Identify the location of the semen samples
2. Open the lid and remove the neck plug.
3. Lift the canister up to frost level inside the neck of the container.
4. Using a pre cooled forceps pick out the straw in 5 to 10 seconds
5. Shake the straw once or twice to remove the liquid nitrogen adhering to the ends.
6. Immediately place the straw in water bath
7. Thawing should be done at 37^0C or minimum of 30 seconds
8. Never return the straw once it was removed from liquid nitrogen.

Procedure for Loading the A.I. Gun

1. Identify the canister from which the desired semen is to be taken
2. Ascertain the colour of the straw by reading of identification tag
3. Remove the lid from the container
4. Lift the proper canister up to the level of the frost line. Never lift the canister above the neck level
5. With a pair of tweezers grasp an individual straw and remove it, at the same time lower the canister immediately back into the container.

If it is not possible to take the straw within 10 seconds, lower the canister back to nitrogen, wait for some time and make next attempt.

6. With wrist movement give one or two jerks to the straw to expel liquid nitrogen trapped at end of factory seal
7. Dip the straw into a clean water bath at 37^0- 40^0C for 30 seconds. During this period the entire straw must be completely submerged in water bath.
8. Remove the straw from water bath and dry the straw with a clean tissue paper or absorbable cotton.
9. Inspect the straw carefully and discard straw with cracks or defective seals. Semen must never come in contact with water.
10. Place the straw in the chamber of insemination gun in such a way that the factory seal should go down
11. To obtain perfect fit with mini straw, it is essential that laboratory seal be removed by cutting at right angle through the middle of the air space. The air space could be brought to the top by gentle tapping of straw.
12. Make sure that the clipped end of straw has a straight clean cut with no jagged edges. Straws cut at other angles or cut too short will result in back flow and wastage of semen at the time of insemination.
13. Fit a sheath over the straw and chamber of the insemination gun and obtain a perfect fit between the extremity of the straw and the cone of the sheath.
14. Move the sheath about 1" up and check whether the straw follows the sheath, if it is not correctly fixed it will not move upwards with the sheath.
15. Fix the sheath by locking the plastic 'O' ring at the flange of the gun with rotating motion. Do not touch the sheath in the tip or middle portion and handle only the base portion.
16. Extrude a tiny drop of semen to remove air bubble, to move the factory seal and to ensure good fitting of the sheath.

The post-thaw survival of spermatozoa is poor after thawing. So, for maximum reproductive efficiency, thawed semen should be used immediately within ten minutes. Therefore, do not thaw more than one straw simultaneously.

❑❑❑

6

Insemination

Insemination of goats may be vaginal, cervical or intrauterine. The methods differ in their complexity and in the expectation of success.

Vaginal insemination using fresh diluted semen is the simplest and quickest method, but generally requires a larger semen dose than the other methods and the success rates reported have been quite variable. Although it cannot be generally recommended, vaginal insemination may be useful where time and resources are limiting factors, or for insemination of maiden females in which the narrow vestibular part of the vagina does not allow full penetration of a speculum.

Cervical insemination using fresh diluted semen is the most commonly used method of artificial insemination of sheep and goats. The equipment used is simple and if adequate personnel are available, large numbers of animals can be inseminated in a short time. When performed properly, cervical insemination of fresh diluted or undiluted semen results in high fertility, comparable with that obtained in standard flock/herd mating. This is the generally recommended method of insemination when fresh diluted or undiluted semen is to be used.

The success rate of cervical insemination using frozen thawed buck semen has been relatively low but satisfactory results can be achieved by repeated inseminations. In some goats intrauterine insemination can be performed through laproscopy. Intrauterine insemination with diluted fresh semen is used when super ovulated females are inseminated in an embryo transfer programme.

Equipment for Vaginal and Cervical AI

The equipment used for vaginal insemination consists simply of a straight plastic pipette connected to a 1.0 ml syringe. It is similar in all respects to that used for cervical insemination, except that the tip is straight instead of being drawn to a crooked point.

The basic equipment for cervical insemination consists of a headlight, a speculum and a pipette. The duck bill type of speculum is preferred to the tubular type since it allows better visibility and location of the cervix and is easier to clean (inside and out) than the latter type. Some specula have a built-in light source. However, a simple medical headlight with a 6-volt bulb and battery is practical for use with the duckbill speculum.

Various pipettes or inseminating guns are used for cervical insemination, but the plastic single-shot disposable pipettes are most popular. These pipettes are constructed of a sturdy but flexible plastic. They are about 30 cm long with about 2.5 mm internal and 4.5 mm external diameter. The opposite end is connected to a 1.0 ml syringe. These pipettes deliver only a single dose at a time. Semi-automatic inseminating devices are not commonly used since it is difficult to clean them and to maintain the semen at the proper temperature before insemination. For cervical insemination of semen packed in straws (liquid or frozen stored semen) a special device called a straw gun is used to discharge the semen from the straw.

Restraint of Does

Insemination should take place in an enclosed shed or barn, which has several pens to facilitate handling of females in groups. It is also advisable to have a Den available for holding the females after insemination. The does should be restrained and presented for insemination in a way which involves minimum time and labour, does not cause unnecessary stress, and which allows quick and efficient location of the insemination site for deposition of semen. The method of restraining the females depends on the facilities available and the method of insemination to be used. In practice, the larger the number of animals to be inseminated the more efficient must be the method of restraint and presentation of the females.

There are several methods used for restraining does for insemination. The method of restraint depends on the method of insemination to be used. The simplest methods are often the most convenient; semi-automatic types of restraining devices are complex and expensive and are not in common use.

Restraint of Females for Vaginal or Cervical Insemination

For vaginal insemination, the females are best restrained in a standing position in a rail or simply confined in a small pen or a race in which they can be held against the side of the pen or race for insemination. The method which allows most convenient presentation of ewes for cervical insemination is often referred to as the over the rail' method. The animal is inclined head downwards over the rail of an inseminating race or pen. It may be more convenient to use a suitable pen for goat does if the are difficult to confine in a race. A portable 'rail crate' may be useful for goats, or when only a few sheep are to be inseminated and other facilities are not available.

The design of an inseminating race should take into account the breed and size of the animals. A wider race and a higher rail are required for larger females than for smaller ones. As a general guide, a convenient rail height for sheep is 85-90 cm with a race width of 60-65 cm. To hold 15-25 females the race should be 6-8 metres long. The race can be constructed on the floor of the shed or elevated off the floor to a more comfortable height for the inseminator. In this case, the whole race should be elevated by about 50 cm. The position of the race should be such that the light from the shed windows is not in front of the inseminator. The females are presented for cervical insemination by an assistant standing in the race and lifting the hindquarters of the animal over the rail while the front legs remain standing on the floor of the race.

Methods of Insemination

Vaginal insemination

Vaginal insemination consists of deposition of semen into the anterior vagina without an attempt to locate the cervix.

The vulva of the female should be wiped with a piece of cotton wool or tissue to avoid contamination of the vagina when introducing the pipette. The pipette is loaded by first withdrawing air to the 0.2 ml mark on the syringe and then drawing up the required dose of semen from a test tube held in a water bath at 37^0 C. The air cushion serves to expel the full volume of semen from the syringe. The pipette is carefully introduced as far as possible into the vagina, sliding the tip along the upper wall to avoid accidental introduction into the urethral orifice on the floor of the vagina. Since a speculum is not normally used, the introduction of the pipette can be facilitated by opening the vulva with the free hand and gently twisting the pipette on entry. The plunger of the syringe is then depressed and the pipette withdrawn.

The inseminating pipette can be re-used several times. Between each insemination it should be properly cleaned with cotton wool or a tissue paper. If a pipette becomes contaminated during insemination, it should be disposed of immediately. To ensure that the pipettes are properly cleaned and dried without interruption to the inseminating procedure, there should be sufficient on hand and an assistant employed solely to clean and re-charge them. It is important that the success of the insemination is not jeopardized by undue haste.

Cervical Insemination

Cervical insemination involves deposition of semen to a depth of up to 3 cm into the cervix. If, as in some animals, the cervix will permit further passage of the pipette, the method can be adapted to become a non-surgical intrauterine insemination.

The 'over the rail' method is most commonly practiced for cervical insemination. The vulva of the doe presented for insemination should be wiped with cotton wool or a tissue paper. The external genitalia of the animals are generally cleaner and the introduction of the speculum is easier and more convenient, when the animals have short wool or hair or when they have been recently crutched.

If a duckbill type of speculum is used it should be inserted into the vagina with its jaws closed and parallel to the lips of the vulva. Excessive force or rough handling of the speculum during insertion may cause injury to the vagina and should be avoided. After the insertion to a depth of 10-13cm, the speculum may be rotated through 90^{0}C (up or down) and its jaws opened. The beam of the headlight it then directed through the open speculum into the anterior vagina. The cervix can be located by gentle manipulation of the speculum sideways or downwards. The jaws of the speculum should not be opened too wide as this may cause pain or stress to the animal. If difficulty is encountered in locating the cervix it is often useful to change the restraining position of the female in case she is in a contorted position.

If any foreign material (such as grass seeds) is observed in the vagina, it should be removed with the aid of a pair of clean long forceps before insemination. When a large amount of mucus has accumulated in the vagina, or when mucus covers the entrance to the cervix, the vagina should be drained. This is done by gently pressing the tip of the speculum against the floor of the vagina, and the closing and withdrawing the speculum. The operation is more efficient when the assistant restraining the ewe or doe lifts her front end so that she drains to the rear more readily.

Some females, particularly those that are susceptible to stress or are roughly handled, may urinate when presented for insemination. If the urine accumulates in the vagina it must be drained and the vagina rinsed with saline, milk or other diluent, or the insemination should be postponed. In this case, the female is placed in a reserve pen and inseminated last.

The inseminating pipette may be loaded by an assistant. To do this, the plunger is first withdrawn to the 0.2 ml mark. The tip of the pipette is then immersed in the semen held in a test tube in a water bath at 30^0C and the appropriate volume of semen drawn up into the pipette.

The inseminator should attempt to introduce the pipette as deep as possible into the cervix without using force. If the pipette penetrates the cervix, semen may be deposited into the uterus by depressing the plunger of the syringe. When the pipette is inserted into the cervix, the speculum should first be slightly withdrawn, and then the semen expelled from the pipette by depressing the plunger of the syringe. Slight withdrawal of the speculum allows closure of the anterior vagina and thereby prevents backflow of semen. After discharge of semen first the pipette and then the speculum are withdrawn from the vagina.

The use of a pipette with an angled tip aids this procedure. Practice is needed to locate the cervix and to introduce the pipette as deeply as possible. In goats, twisting of the pipette may be necessary to achieve deep penetration of the cervix or intrauterine insemination. Complete penetration of the cervix can be felt quite easily by the lack of resistance to penetration of the pipette, but care should be taken to avoid pushing the pipette in too deep as this may cause damage to the wall of the uterus.

Kidding rates in relation to depth of cervical insemination in crossbred Angora does

Depth of cervical insemination	No. of does kidded per inseminated (%)			
	Fresh diluted semen		Frozen-thawed semen	
Up to 1 cm	37/88	(42.0%)	17/63	(27.0%)
1.0 to 3.0 cm	74/127	(58.3%)	39/85	(45.9%)
Into uterus	56/81	(69.1%)	7/102	(68.6%)

It has been shown in both sheep and goats that increasing the depth of semen deposition into the cervix result in higher fertility.

With regard to the potential depth of insemination in goat does, there is individual animal variation, between-herd variation, and probably some differences due to the phenotype of inseminating pipette used and the skill of the operator. In general, the cervix can be penetrated and semen deposited into the uterus in 30-50% of does. It is interesting to note that animals in which the cervix is penetrated at one insemination do not necessarily have a penetrable cervix at a subsequent insemination.

To prevent the spread of disease, it is important that the instruments are cleaned between each insemination. The interior and exterior jaws of the speculum should be cleaned thoroughly by wiping them with cotton wool moistened with alcohol. The speculum should be dry before use on the next animal. When care is taken to ensure that the inseminating pipettes are not contaminated with urine or faeces they can be used for several inseminations. Between each insemination, the pipette must be wiped with piece of cotton wool or tissue. It is important that the pipette is clean and dry before re-introducing it to the semen pool. Any contamination may kill the spermatozoa in the semen.

After insemination the ewes and does should be released into a covered or shaded yard, or preferably into a pen in the shed, where they can remain undisturbed for at least 2-3 hours after insemination.

Time of Insemination

For successful artificial insemination, some knowledge of the length of oestrus and time of ovulation is required so that the time of insemination can be adjusted accordingly. In most does ovulation occurs at a fixed time in relation to the onset of oestrus.

The volume and physical state of the vagino-cervical mucus changes during the course of oestrus, and these characteristics can be sued as a guide for determining the stage of between mucus traits and fertility, and the optimum time for insemination is when the mucus is copious and clear to slightly cloudy. However, accurate determination of the time of onset of oestrus and optimum time for insemination under practical conditions is problematic. Synchronization of oestrus makes the time of ovulation predictable.

The time of insemination caries according to the method of insemination used. In general, vaginal insemination is used for females in natural or synchronized oestrus, and synchronization is necessary for intrauterine insemination.

Time of insemination of females in natural oestrus (vaginal or cervical AI)

For vaginal and cervical Al the inseminations is most successful if it is done before ovulation, but close to its occurrence. In general, the optimum time for insemination of does is 12-18 hours after the onset of oestrus.

When females in natural oestrus are to be inseminated, oestrus is usually detected by teaser males. Association with males may affect the duration of oestrus; oestrus is generally shorter and ovulation may occur earlier in females run continuously with males than in those 'hand teased'. When marked (oestrous) females are drafted only once daily (morning) they should be inseminated soon after drafting. When two daily drafting (morning and evening) are done, the evening-drafted females should be inseminated first the next morning, followed by the morning-drafted females. Twice-daily drafting increases the number of females detected in oestrus by 15-20% and insemination can be timed more accurately in relation to ovulation.

Time of ovulation in synchronized oestrus (cervical or intrauterine AI)

When oestrus has been synchronized there is no need to detect oestrus with teaser males; insemination can be performed at a fixed time in relation to the synchronization treatment. The time of ovulation varies slightly between individuals, with season, and with the use of PMSG or the male effect to stimulate oestrus and ovulation. However, ovulation occurs within close limits of most animals. If progestogen pessary is used in conjunction with PMSG and 5-10% teaser males, the majority of females will be in oestrus within 36-48 hours and ovulate about 60 hours after pessary withdrawal. The insemination times recommended below apply to this method of synchronization of oestrus and ovulation; other methods may require slight modification of the times.

1. Cervical insemination

As with females in natural oestrus, insemination should take place before, but close to, ovulation. The optimum time for insemination is between 48 and 58 hours (generally a single insemination at 55 hours) after pessary withdrawal.

2. Intrauterine insemination

Manipulation of the reproductive tract close to the time of ovulation may interfere with the successful transfer of ovulated ova from the ovary to the oviduct and this time should be avoided for intrauterine insemination.

Frozen-thawed buck semen is generally used with intrauterine insemination. In this case, the optimum time for semen deposition in does is 60-66 hours after pessary withdrawal.

Superovulated females, treated with relatively larger doses of gonadotrophin, ovulate earlier than normal. Such females are generally inseminated with large doses of fresh spermatozoa (at least 100 million motile). In this case, intrauterine insemination may be performed 36-48 hours after pessary withdrawal. When frozen-thawed semen is used in superovulated females, intrauterine insemination should be performed 44-48 hours after pessary withdrawal.

Number of Inseminations within One Oestrus

Under field conditions females are usually inseminated only once during oestrus. To increase fertility, two inseminations can be performed within one oestrus. The effect of double insemination varies depending on the time of the first insemination in relation to ovulation (or time of sponge removal). For ewes and does in natural oestrus, the increase in fertility to double insemination is more evident when the first insemination occurs early in oestrus than when it occurs in mid to late oestrus. In practice, double insemination guards against the possibility that one insemination may be performed too early in relation to ovulation. For females in synchronized oestrus, double insemination is performed at 48-50 and 58-60 hours after pessary withdrawal. When females are in natural oestrus, the first insemination is performed soon after drafting and the second one 8-12 hours later.

Double insemination within one oestrus is, however, recommended when liquid-stored and frozen-thawed semen is used for cervical insemination. Double insemination is not recommended when intrauterine insemination is performed, either by laparoscopy or via the cervix in goats.

Dos of inseminate

The recommended minimum numbers of spermatozoa are important ones. When double vaginal or cervical insemination is performed, the recommended dose should be used at each insemination.

Steps for vaginal or cervical insemination

i) Use clean, dry and sterile pipettes with smooth, non-abrasive ends.

ii) Connect each pipette to a 1.0 ml syringe and ensure that it works smoothly. Lubricate the plunger with vaseline, if necessary.

iii) Prepare paper tissue or cotton wool piece for wiping and cleaning the pipettes.

iv) Prepare separate pieces of cotton wool for wiping the vulva of the female and the speculum between inseminations.

v) For cervical insemination fix the headlight in place and connect to the battery.

vi) Aspirate 0.2 ml of air followed by the required volume of semen, which is kept in a water bath at 30^0 C, into the pipette (preferably done by an assistant)

vii) When the female is presented for insemination, preferably over a rail for cervical insemination or in a standing position for vaginal insemination, wipe the vulva with cotton wool.

viii) Introduce the speculum carefully into the vagina of the female (10-13 cm) and locate the cervix.

ix) Observe the type and amount of mucus in the vagina and drain if necessary.

x) Introduce the pipette as far as possible into the cervix. A twisting motion may be sued but do not use force.

xi) Withdraw the speculum slightly and press the plunger of the syringe to expel the semen.

xii) Withdraw the pipette and then the speculum from the vagina

xiii) For vaginal insemination introduce the pipette through the lips of the vulva and gently push to the anterior vagina. Push the plunger to expel the semen and then withdraw the pipette.

xiv) Clean the inseminating pipette with tissue or cotton wool. Ensure it is dry before re-use. Do not re-use dirty or contaminated pipettes.

xv) Wipe the speculum with cotton wool moistened with alcohol and dry by wiping with a tissue paper before inseminating the next female.

xvi) Release the inseminated females into a shaded yard, or into a pen in the shed, and allow them to remain undisturbed for at least 2-3 hours after insemination. Avoid rough handling and the use of aggressive dogs at all times.

❑❑❑

7

Management of Does after Insemination

The management of does after AI does not differ greatly from that of animals bred naturally. A knowledge on basic husbandry principles, particularly with regard to nutrition, health and management during pregnancy, parturition and lactation, is assumed and is beyond the scope of this. However, normal husbandry practice may need modification specifically for an Al program, and this is discussed below.

Re-breeding of Female, which Fail to Conceive to Artificial Insemination

The proportion of females, which conceive, depends on several factors but will not usually exceed 75%. However, females, which do not conceive to AI, re-bred at a subsequent oestrus in order to achieve a higher overall lambing/kidding rate. This is possible if the AI program is performed in the breeding season. Females in which oestrus and ovulation has been artificially stimulated in the non-breeding season will not usually continue to cycle.

Re-breeding by A.I.

Re-breeding of females by AI requires the use of teaser males with harnesses and crayons to detect oestrus. If the female did not conceive to AI, oestrus will occur after about 19-21 days in most goats (one oestrus cycle length). However, to detect females with shorter cycles, the teasers should be introduced 10-12 days after AI, ensuring that the color of the crayon has been changed from that used previously. About 2% teasers are used for a non-synchronized flock or herd and 3-4% when the females have been synchronized at the previous cycle. In the later case most non-pregnant females can be expected to show oestrus over a 4-5 day period. The females may be drafted once or twice daily for insemination.

Re-breeding by Natural Mating

In this case, intact males may be introduced to the females 10-12 days after AI. About 2% males are used when the females have not been previously synchronized, and 3-4% when they have been synchronized at the previous cycle. It is not necessary to use harnesses and crayons on the males unless it is proposed to keep records of the number of females returning to service.

Whatever method of re-breeding is used it is important that the time of lambing/kidding is carefully recorded. Those animals, which conceived to AI, will give birth in less than 155 days from the time of insemination; those, which conceived to subsequent re-breeding, will give birth more than 160 days after the original AI.

Although females subsequently detected in oestrus are unlikely to have conceived to the original AI, the converse may not be true, that is females, which do not return to service, are not necessarily pregnant. The proportion of females, which return to service, is an early, but not very reliable, indication of the success of AI.

Pregnancy Diagnosis

Diagnosis of pregnancy aids flock/herd management. If it is known which females are not pregnant they can be separated from the breeding flock/herd and re-bred. The pregnant once may also be afforded the best pastures.

Apart from the unreliable 'return to service' method, there are several methods of pregnancy diagnosis in goats. These included assay of blood hormones, ultra sonic techniques, and laparoscopy. Some methods of pregnancy diagnosis require that the breeding date be precisely known. At present there is no cheap and reliable method capable of detecting pregnancy before 17-20 days. Pregnancy diagnosis is not widely used in goats.

Management During Pregnancy

Since AI involves considerable time and effort, the success of the operation should not be jeopardized due to neglect of the requirements of the pregnant females. No matter what the method of breeding, some embryonic and foetal losses are inevitable. However, poor results are often due to bad management of pregnant females, or adverse environmental factors and not due to factors related to AI itself.

The management of females in an AI program is basically similar to that of those bred naturally but since the time of insemination is known precisely, management can be better controlled. This is particularly true for females in which oestrus has been synchronized as they can be treated as a group. Normal management procedures require that the best pasture is reserved for females in the last trimester of pregnancy and during lactation when the nutritional demands are highest. This should be considered when planning an AI program. It is also important that females are in good condition at the time of insemination and for the first third of pregnancy when the placenta is developing rapidly. Temperature stress (40-45^{0}C) in the first trimester of pregnancy may adversely affect placental development and subsequently, the growth of the foetus. To avoid embryonic and foetal losses due to pathological factors prophylactic measures should be strictly observed.

Management During Parturition

Since the date of insemination is known, the time of parturition (lambing/kidding) can be predicted. The length of gestation in goats varies slightly with breed, age of dam, and the number and sex of fetuses. Average gestation length is close to 149 days in goats (range 143-155 days)

When insemination is closely synchronized management of parturition can be simplified. Several reports have shown that supervision of parturition in small paddocks or barns can reduce neonatal losses, that losses occurring during or shortly after birth, to less than 3% (losses may reach 20% under range kidding). Closely synchronized births also facilitate cross fostering of orphan lambs or kids. However, it should also be noted that synchronized flocks or herds are particularly susceptible to heavy neonatal losses due to freak climatic conditions occurring coincidentally with the peak time of parturition.

When the time of insemination is known, and pregnancy has been confirmed, parturition may be slightly advanced, or synchronized, by drug or hormone treatment close to the expected time of birth. This is sometime practiced in intensive husbandry systems, for example those in France, but is not common elsewhere.

❑❑❑

8

Factors Influencing Fertility after Artificial Insemination

In an AI program, if the animals are healthy, in good condition, and free of abnormalities of the reproductive tract, there are a number of factors, which may influence the results. These are listed below:

1. Number of spermatozoa

The number of normal, viable spermatozoa inseminated below a minimum limit affects fertility. The number required varies according to the storage state (fresh, liquid-stored or frozen-thawed) and the site of insemination.

2. Method and technique of insemination

Fertility varies with the method of insemination. Intrauterine insemination (by laparoscopy via the cervix) is more successful than cervical insemination, particularly for frozen semen. For vaginal insemination only fresh semen should be used and females should not be synchronized with pharmacological agents. Increasing depth of cervical insemination improves fertility.

3. Time of insemination

Insemination too early or too late in relation to ovulation is detrimental to fertility. The time of insemination is more critical when liquid-stored or frozen-thawed rather than fresh semen is used since stored spermatozoa have a shorter viable period in the female reproductive tract. Females with a short oestrus may have reduced fertility.

4. Type of oestrus (natural or controlled)

Fertility of sheep after cervical insemination is often lower when pharmaceutical agents have synchronized oestrus, though this problem can be overcome by use of exogenous gonadotrophins or intrauterine insemination. In goats, there is little influence of synchronization on fertility. The type and level of treatment with pharmacological agents can affect fertility.

5. Age of females

Fertility is generally lower in young or primiparous animals than in mature animals.

6. Season of treatment

Fertility is usually lower when animals are inseminated outside the normal breeding season.

7. Stress factors

Careless or rough handling of females at insemination or in the period of establishment of pregnancy affects fertility.

8. Embryonic and foetal mortality

Environmental and nutritional stress or diseases during pregnancy may result in embryonic or foetal mortality. Placental insufficiency or in goats particularly, failure of the corpus luteum of pregnancy, may result in abortion.

9. Hygiene

Careless handling or contamination of equipment may result in a reduction in viability, of spermatozoa or spread diseases of the reproductive tract.

It is important to note that when disappointing results are obtained, the AI technology itself is- unlikely to be at fault. The fault will almost certainly be found in (i) improper application of that technology (ii) improper management, or (iii) environmental factors.

❑❑❑

9

Recording of Data

Recording of data during an AI program is necessary for the assessment of the success and value of the technique. Records of the semen characteristics of individual sires, and of the females inseminated with their semen, should be made at the time of insemination. These data can then be compared with the records of births to obtain an overall assessment of the performance of individual sires.

Records of births can be kept for groups of females or in the case of goat studs, for individual females. The recording should be done as soon as possible after kidding. Delayed recording fails to account for any kids which may be lost between birth and time of recording, for example due to adverse climatic conditions or other reasons not associated with AI program. Records can be made at parturition if this is supervised, or otherwise 7-10 days afterwards to allow time for bonding of mothers and their new born. Note that identification of individual kids in a group is very difficult at the latter stage, so stud breeders should be prepared to supervise 'parturition or keep the pregnant females in individual confinement at this time.

The proper way of expressing the results of an AI program is the percentage of females giving birth of the total number inseminated. When the number of newborn is recorded at birth, the percentage of kids born of the number of females giving birth can also be calculated; this provides information on twinning or multiple births. In some areas, the kidding percentage is defined as the number of kids born of the total number of females in the group.

Examples of the calculation are

1. Kidding percentage (females giving birth to females inseminated)

Number of females inseminated = 800

Number of females giving birth = 568

$$\text{Kidding percentage} = \frac{568 \times 100}{800} = 71.0\%$$

2. Kidding percentage (kids born to females inseminated)

Number of females inseminated = 800

Number of kids born = 650

$$\text{Kidding percentage} = \frac{650 \times 100}{800} = 81.3\%$$

3. Multiple (or twinning) rate (Kids born to females giving birth)

Number of females giving birth = 568

Number of kids born = 650

$$\text{Percentage of kids born} = \frac{650 \times 100}{568} = 114.4\%$$

❑❑❑

10

Maintenance of Cryogenic Containers

The liquid nitrogen refrigerators are constructed in such a way that the three pathways of heat transfer, conduction, convection and radiation, are minimised. Creating a super vacuum prevents the transfer of heat through conduction and convection. Therefore the liquid nitrogen refrigerator is a double walled container, the space between the walls is evacuated of air. Winding the inner vessel alternatively with paper and foil prevents the radiation. The inner vessel is connected with the outer vessel with glue it is not supported by a strong welding. Hence, the neck is the weakest part of the whole refrigerator and sudden tipping on one side will cause damage to the neck.

Safety Aspects in Handling Cryogenic Agents

There are a number of general precautions and safe practices, to be observed because of two important properties of cryogenic fluid; they are extremely cold and very small amount of liquid is converted into very large amount of gas. When liquid nitrogen evaporates into gaseous form, it occupies 700 times its volume.

Safe handling of liquid nitrogen

- Liquid nitrogen should be handled carefully as it can produce 'frost bite' on the skin similar to burn, even if it is in contact for more than a few seconds.
- The vapour of liquid nitrogen is also cold and can produce cold burns. Cold vapour can damage delicate tissues such as eyes even if exposed for a short period.
- One should not look into an open liquid nitrogen container without eye protection.

- Boiling and splashing always occur when filling up a warm container. Always perform these operations **slowly** to minimize boiling and splashing and keep your eyes away from the container.
- Always use stainless steel tongs with long handles to remove any object immersed in liquid nitrogen. Loose fitting gloves made of woolen, asbestos or leather can be used for handling. Cold metal may stick to skin and tear the flesh when attempts are made to withdraw the cold object from bare hands or fingers. Specially made Cryo-gloves are also available for this purpose.
- Care should be taken to avoid spilling of liquid nitrogen into shoes.
- Use containers specifically designed to hold liquid nitrogen. All containers have vent or safety device to allow the escape of nitrogen vapour. Inadequate venting or closing tightly can result in excessive gas pressure, which can damage or burst a container. Use only the stopper supplied by the firm; never plug the containers tightly.

Care of liquid nitrogen containers

The cryogenic containers are double walled vessels, with annular space evacuated and sealed. In addition, several types of insulation *viz.*, vacuum alone, expanded foam, gas filled powder and fibrous material, evacuated powder or evacuated super insulation are used as thermal insulators. The outer walls of containers are made of stainless steel, carbon steel or aluminium alloys.

- Extreme care should be exercised in handling containers.
- The cryogenic equipment is specific and they are meant to store only the particular liquid for which they are made.
- Welding or piercing the container wall is dangerous.
- Keep the container always in upright position.
- Protect the container against shock and rough handling. During transport support the container with soft padding (rubber, thermocole, wooden crates *etc.*).
- Protect against direct sunlight and hot blowing winds.
- Charging of warm container should be slow.
- Avoid frequent cooling and warming of containers. Thermal stress may cause so much strain within it that the inner wall of container may crack. Appearance of moisture on the outer wall of container is

a sign of damaged container. Do not dry the container meant for regular use.

- Find out the evaporation rate for each Container, so that the periodicity of topping could be organized.
- When the vacuum disappears, the insulating capacity is lost. Repairing of damaged containers has to be done by the manufacturer only. Hence, containers should be handled very gently particularly during transport in vehicles.

Assessment of liquid nitrogen level

The evaporation rate of liquid nitrogen varies between containers (even among the same make and capacity), temperature of the room in which it is stored and number of times it is opened. Hence, periodic checking of the level of the liquid nitrogen is essential. The minimum level of liquid nitrogen should keep the straws completely submerged in liquid nitrogen.

To measure the level, take a 'dipstick' (slender stick made of wood or metal) and gently lower it into the container and rest it at the bottom. Hollow tube should not be used. After5-1O seconds, take it out and wave in the air. The atmospheric air condenses as a 'frost' on the dipstick to the level of liquid nitrogen. Read the level, 1 cm below the end of frost Line (giving allowance for boiling of liquid nitrogen when the dipstick was inserted). By using the calibration chart, the volume of nitrogen can also be estimated. However, frequent measuring leads to unnecessary evaporation of liquid nitrogen.

Liquid nitrogen has a specific gravity of 0.82. i.e., one litre weighs 0.82 kg (1 kg = 1.22 litres). Based on weight, the quantity of liquid nitrogen in litres could be calculated. For this purpose, the weight of the empty container should also be known.

❑❑❑

11

Cleaning of Utensils

All utensils and instruments used for collection, handling of semen and for insemination should be thoroughly cleaned and sterilized. Dirty or improperly cleaned equipment can be highly detrimental to an Al program. For washing equipment, tap water or clean rainwater should be used. A solution of laboratory glassware detergent (for example, Pyroneg, 7X, or others) in water should be used at the concentration recommended by the manufacturer. It is best to allow the equipment to soak for 1-2 hours in the detergent before scrubbing clean, It is important that all equipment such as artificial vaginas, collecting glasses and pipettes be immersed in water or detergent immediately after use to avoid contaminating substances becoming encrusted.

To clean utensils with open surfaces, brushes of the appropriate size should be used with a solution of the detergent in warm water. Pipettes should be soaked before rinsing with several changes of water, preferably under pressure by blowing and sucking, or in an automatic pipette washer if available. After washing, all equipment should be thoroughly rinsed with several changes of water to remove all traces of the detergent first with the tap or rain water and then with several changes of distilled water. After shaking off excess water the equipment may be dried in an incubator or air-dryer.

Sterilization of equipment is essential. The glassware can be heat sterilized, possibly contained in a stainless steel sterilizing box, in an oven. The glassware should be brought to a temperature of at least 165° C and maintained at this temperature for at least 1 hour. The instruments can be kept in the sealed sterilizing box until use. Alternatively, each item can be wrapped tightly in aluminium foil (before sterilization) for protection. Glass pipettes should be sterilized this way. Plastic pipettes are sterilized with 70 % alcohol; after soaking in the alcohol for about an hour, the pipettes should be placed in a pipette holder or wrapped in clean paper or aluminium foil where they can be left to allow the excess alcohol to evaporate. Before using the pipettes, they should- be thoroughly rinsed with isotonic diluent (or sterile 0.9% saline) to remove all traces of the alcohol before use. Extreme care should be taken when cleaning and sterilizing equipment during use, for example, the speculum and inseminating pipettes during insemination. The speculum should be wiped with cotton wool moistened with 70% alcohol and care taken to ensure that it is thoroughly dry before use on another animal. Because of the danger of killing spermatozoa by contact with disinfectants or sterilizing solutions, it is not recommended that pipettes are sterilized between each insemination. They should be wiped clean with cotton wool or a tissue and discarded if they become contaminated in any way.

In order to protect the clean utensils and instruments from dust, insects or other contaminants, they should be placed in a clean cupboard or other suitable container.

12

Equipment Required for An Artificial Insemination Program

Vaginal and cervical insemination

i) Liquid Nitrogen semen storage containers

ii) Liquid Nitrogen transport containers

iii) Water bath

iv) An appropriate restraining device, rail, pen or race for presentation of females for insemination

v) Speculum, preferably the duck-bill type, about 15 cm long, opening to about 6-7 cm. a smaller one may be necessary for young females

vi) Headlight with 6-volt bulb and 2-3 spare bulbs

vii) 6-volt batteries (3-4)

viii) Inseminating pipettes (allow one for every 5-10 females)

ix) 1 ml plastic calibrated syringes with tube to connect to inseminating pipette (6-10)

x) 'Straw gun' or 'pistolet' if straws are used.

Multipurpose and other glassware

i) Oven for sterilizing glassware

ii) Table - 2 Nos.

iii) Bench covering (clean paper, plastic or cloth)

iv) Cloths/dust covers for instruments

v) Instrument holding cupboard

vi) Thermometers (°C) (3-4)

vii) Racks for test tubes and collecting glasses

viii) Stainless steel forceps, 25-30 cm

ix) Pasteur pipettes (washed and sterilized) and teats

x) Brushes (2 cm and 7 cm diameter) for cleaning glassware and artificial vaginas

xi) Several plastic buckets and bowls for washing up

xii) Towels and cloths

xiii) Scissors

xiv) Plastic wash (squeeze) bottles

xv) Electrical extension cables and double adaptors

xvi) Ear tags and applicators

xvii) Notebook(s)

xviii) Pens and/or pencils

xix) Indelible (waterproof) marker pens for glassware

xx) Small general tool kit for minor repair of equipment

xxi) Brooms and garbage bins

xxii) Protective clothing; boots and overalls

Disposable items

i) Laboratory detergent

ii) General sterilizing/antiseptic solution

iii) 70% alcohol in glass distilled water

iv) Glass-distilled water for rinsing glassware and instruments

v) A supply of tap or rain water

vi) Soap

vii) Paper towels

viii) Aluminium foil

ix) Paper tissues

x) Cotton wool

xi) Carbage bags

Name and addresses of suppliers of A.I. equipment for goats

1. IMV Technologies
   IMV India Private Limited
   Plot No. 747, Phase - V
   Udyog Vihar
   Gurgaon - 122 016
   Haryana State
   www.imv-technoloqies.com
   Phone: 0124 4004430

2. IBP Division
   Southern Warehouse
   Visfotak Bhavan
   161, Greams Road
   Chennai - 600 006
   Phone: 044 28278353

3. Jayanth Brothers
   425-A, Kilpauk Garden Road
   Chennai - 600 010
   e-mail: jayanthbros@eth.net
   Phone: 044 26447043
   044 26461736

□□□

PART-II :
ARTIFICIAL INSEMINATION IN SHEEP

13

Introduction

Artificial insemination (A.I.) technique in sheep is relatively less developed as compared to cattle and buffaloes. The-main obstacles to the widespread use of A.I. in sheep are lack of overt signs of oestrus and narrow and tortuos cervical canal of the uterus in ewes. On the male side, significant decline in fertility is observed with the use of chilled semen after 6 hours of storage, though the spermatozoa still maintain acceptable motility. With frozen semen, the successful revival of spermotozoa after deep freezing is not accompanied by full fertility as it is in the bull.

Despite these constraints, there is an urgent need for introduction of A.I. in sheep using frozen semen. Crossbreeding is gaining importance as a tool to improved productivity per animal. However, exotic sheep will not stand the rigours of the village and tropical environment. They have to be kept in most comfortable environment in selected locations and the village flocks have to be bred with frozen semen. Frozen semen has its advantage even in pure breeding as it facilitates avoidance of inbreeding and genetic drift in purebred stocks, making it possible to operate with small numbers. Preservation of germ plasm in the form of frozen semen is the best, safe, cheap and quick method. Even the extinct breed can be regenerated through the use of frozen semen. Through 5 generations of repeated back crossing 97 per cent of the inheritance of rare breed gets established. Research in the field of A.I. in sheep has been very active in many laboratories in the recent past.

❑❑❑

14

Semen Collection

Selection of Rams

Generally there is little scope for selection in exotic breeds as the nucleus flocks are most often small. Hence under those circumstances sex libido and semen quality would at best be the criteria for selection of rams. If selection is possible, it is based on four important traits of productivity – number of lambs born, weaning weight, weight at 6 months of age and fleece weight at 12 months of age. The first trait is mandatory for all users, while others are optional. The criteria used are weaning and 6 months weight for meat breeds while for dual purpose breeds all four traits are used. They may be combined into an aggregate index and used. When selection is for weaning weight it should be adjusted for the effects of age at weaning, type of birth and age of dam.

The simplest way to adjust weaning weight for age of lamb at weaning is to calculate a regression of weaning weight on age and to use this for the correction. Alternately, plot the weaning weight on age on a graph sheet, draw the best straight line possible through the points and use the slope of the line to correct for the ages of the lambs. To adjust for the - type of birth, the classes considered will be single, twin and twin raised as single. The age of dam effects may be considered by classifying ewes into 2, 3 and 4 to 6 year-old ewes. Since this effect is most marked between 2 year-old and older ewes, separation of dams into these two categories is often adequate, particularly in small flocks. Correction factors for adjusting the age corrected weaning weight for' type of birth and age of dam can be obtained by the method of fitting constants. However, when the trait selected is 6 months weight, adjustments are unnecessary as this weight is not much influenced by the above factors. The body weight at weaning is less heritable than the body weight at later ages. In the tropics animals are rarely slaughtered at weaning. Hence body weights at later ages with their high heritability are more important than weaning weight.

Greasy fleece weight is simple to measure and has high heritability and a high genetic correlation with clean fleece weight. The important traits of wool quality are fibre diameter (finer for apparel, coarser for carpet wool), staple length (a minimum desirable length for both), per cent medullated fibres (low or zero for apparel, essential to a certain extent for carpet wool), kemp (preferably completely absent for both) and fibre strength (no tender spots along the staple). The above fibre qualifies are measured on a sample from the mid-side. The most important among them are fibre diameter and per cent medullation.

Among the section objectives for sheep, reproductive rate has higher priority in all systems of sheep production. Reproductive rate can be increased either by raising the number of offspring at a parturition or by decreasing the period between parturitions. In tropical countries, where breeding seasons are long and nutritional level frequently low, the latter may be the more practical course, as a dam might find difficulty in rearing more than one lamb. Where multiple births are considered, the simplest way is to select rams from among multiple-born lambs on the basis of other criteria such as growth rate and wool weight.

Training of Rams

The prospective sires should be given special ration in addition to grazing. If young males are separated from females, they should be introduced to females at least of rams can be started around one year of age. Ewes in oestrus can be mixed with young rams so that they will show interest in females and attempt mounting. The young rams are handled frequently by the person collecting semen (particularly during feeding concentrates). He remains near the rams during mounting and touches the sheath to get rid of shyness on their part. In very timid rams a few natural service can be allowed initially. Subsequently, when artificial vagina (A.V) is applied such rams do not mind the presence of strangers. Oestrus can be induced in culled ewes by injecting 125 mg of cloprostenol intramuscularly once in 3 or 4 days. Immense patience is required on the part of the operator to observe the idiosyncracies of the rams and train them properly. It is advisable to introduce the rams to ewes in oestrus for short duration several times rather than allowing for longer time, less frequently.

Indigenous and crossbred rams are easier to train than exotic rams. Exotic rams start showing libido around 1½ years and the failure rate may be as high as 50 percent. Better feeding and management may help alleviate this problem to some extent.

Collection of Semen

In Wolly breeds, it is better to shear the wool in the region between scrotum and prepuce to get a better view of the penis during collection. The artificial vagina method of collection is easy to perform; but it requires a ewe in oestrus. The A.V. consists of a thick cylindrical rubber hose (20 cm x 5 cm) and a latex liner (30 cm) to be fitted inside (Fig. 2.1). Both ends of the latex liner are rolled inwards and fitted on to the hose tightly without folds or wrinkles. It may be secured more tightly on either ends with rubber bands from discarded liners. Fitting of a collection cup completes the assembling of A.V. Rubber cone for ejaculation and diverting the flow of semen is not necessary as most of the semen is ejaculated into the graduated (0.1 ml accuracy) collection cup.

Hot water (50° to 70°C) is poured into the A.V. after unscrewing the metal valve. The temperature of the AV. should be between 41° and 45°C which can be checked with a clean mercury thermometer. It is advisable to use lower temperature of the range for young rams. Adult and older rams may require higher temperature of the A.V. The temperature of hot water amount of hot water and air are adjusted in such a way that the required temperature of the A.V. is obtained. Using a sterile glass rod (6 mm dia.) with round end, liquid paraffin is applied at the entrance up to a. depth of 5 cm. The collection cup is kept in the incubator at 37°C and fitted just before collection. Now the A.V. is ready for collection and must be held at an angle of 450 to 500 down so that the hot water keeps the temperature of the A.V. at the entrance. (Fig. 2.2)

Collection yard having a service crate must be near the window of the laboratory, so that minimum time elapses between collection and keeping it in the water bath at 30°C. A ewe in oestrus or a teaser ram (for trained rams) is secured in a service crate. The ram meant for collection is let loose under the supervision of an attendant. In young ram it is advisable to apply the A.V. when it mounts and makes searching movements of the penis. If it is prevented from mounting to give false mounts, the act may frighten them. In fully trained rams one or two false mounts may be allowed without upsetting their libido. Giving false mounts before collection has the beneficial effects of improving volume and quality of semen collected. Merino rams, generally, have shorter reaction time and hence two false mounts may result in ejaculation outside the A.V. For rams with shorter reaction time they can be held in the presence of a ewe for about 5 minutes and then collection made. GeneralIy lack of libido and reduced libido are overcome if the collections are made in the presence of rams waiting for collection.

When the ram mounts with fully erected penis, it is directed into the A.V. by gently touching the sheath. Quick reflexes are essential on the part of the operator to avoid difficulties in collection. The penis should not be touched while directing it. At the time of ejaculation the ram makes a strong forward and upward thrust and then dismounts. After ejaculation, the A.V. is held vertically so that all the semen is drained into the collection cup which is then transfered to the laboratory for processing. The ram should not be suddenly withdrawn from the ewe after collection. It is allowed to remain with the ewe for a few minutes and then removed.

The frequency of collection depends on the age and libido of rams. In young rams one or two collections may be made every week. In older rams, semen may be collected daily for 3 or 4 days followed by a rest of 2 days. Generally, regular collection of semen can be made around 2 years and continued upto 5 years of age. If daily collections are made the volume of semen may be reduced; but there may not be any reduction in other quality attributes. When the semen is used for freezing, first ejaculate collected after 4 or 5 days rest has to be discarded to ensure better freezing. If two collections are made in quick succession in a day, the second ejaculate is generally found to have better motility and freerzability.

❑❑❑

15

Semen Evaluation

Before introducing a ram to AI programme (chilled semen or frozen storage) the quality of semen must be assessed properly. The overall judgement may be based on 2 or 3 ejaculates taken on different days. In practice, the first 2 or 3 collections are discarded and subsequent semen samples are used for quality assessment. Normally, volume, colour, consistency, mass activity, progressively motile spermatozoa after dilution, live and dead count and abnormal count are recorded in semen samples immediately after collection.

Volume

Volume of the ejaculate can be directly read from the graduated collection cup. If accurate measurements are needed, finely graduated 1 or 2 ml serological pipettes can be used. Volume of semen varies between 0.5 and 1.5 ml with an average of 1.0 ml. It varies even within rams in successive ejaculates. Younger rams produce lesser volume than older ones. Around 2 years of age the volume reaches its maximum. Adequate prestimulation and false mounts and periodical sexual rest will help harvest larger volume of semen.

Colour and Consistency

Colour and consistency vary from milky to thick creamy. Except in young rams, semen of milky consistency is pot fit for AI work. Semen of thin creamy consistency is not diluted more than 1:1.

Mass Activity

Mass activity of semen is estimated immediately after collection by placing a thick drop of semen on a warm (37°C) microscopic slide without a cover slip and examining at the low power magnification (50x/100x). Wave motion characteristics or swirl motion of the spermatozoa are recorded in 0 to 5 scale. When the mass activity is highest (score 5), dense rapidly moving waves and eddies are noticed. In such samples individual spermatozoa cannot be observed because of their quick movement within the field of observation. In the next lower grade (score 4), vigorous movement of speramatozoa is noticed but the eddies and waves are not so rapid as for score 5. Semen samples having less mass activity than 4 are not suitable for AI work. When the semen is in short supply as in the case of exotic rams, samples with score 3 can be used with reservation under low dilution ratio (1:1 or 1:2) as freshly diluted semen. However, such samples are unfit for frozen storage.

Estimation of Progressively Motile Spermatozoa

This is one subjective test which has been used extensively for research and in routine A.I. work. The motility test is used to assess the quality of diluted semen, stored or frozen-thawed semen. Motility is easy to observe but difficult to explain in objective units of measurement.

A small drop of semen (discharged through a capillary tube of small bore) is placed on clean grease-free, warm (37°C) slide and covered with a round or square clean cover slip (19 mm). It should be ensured that the drop is spread uniformly due to capillary action and not due to pressing of the cover slip. The use of cover slip provides a uniform film, restricts floating of sperm cells and delays drying of the smear. In cold climate a warm stage should be used in the microscope to maintain the temperature. The operator should scan several fields on the slide at the high power magnification (400x) of microscope and the field with highest motility should be chosen. The proportion (percentage) of progressively motile spermatozoa (i.e. moving in forward direction) is estimated in these areas. Since the estimation of motility is subjective, the values are generally expressed in grades of 10 (eg. 60, 70, 80 percent etc.) and occasionally in multiples of 5 (eg. 40, 45, 50 percent etc.).

Certain precautions are to be taken while examining the motility of diluted or frozen-thawed semen. The motility test involves handling of living cells which are sensitive to extrinsic influences. These might destroy the sperm cell, impair or alter their motility. Semen samples should be protected against admixture of water, chemicals and solutions that are not isotonic to sperm. The final opinion about motility should not be based on single estimation unless the test indicated higher motile cells. Lower values should be checked by re-examination of semen with extreme care to avoid technical errors. A good semen sample diluted after collection should have more than 70 to 80 per cent progressively motile spermatozoa.

Concentration

Concentration is estimated for research purposes using a haemocytometer. As the concentration of the ram semen is high (2,000 to 5,000 million/ml), neat semen is sucked into the RBC pipette upto 0.2 mark and the rest of the procedure is similar to that of cattle semen. The final figures are multiplied by 2.5 to get the concentration per ml. Formal saline or 3% saline solution is used for immobilising the spermatozoa.

Photoelectric colorimeter method is the fastest and more reliable method of estimating sperm concentration. It is as accurate as the mean of two or three haemocytometer counts. It measures the amount of a beam of standard light that is deflected and absorbed by a standard volume of semen diluted at a standard rate. Each colorimeter must be calibrated against diluted semen of known concentration as determined by the haemocytometer method.

Preparation of calibration chart

i) Choose a red filter at a wave length of 640 nm.

ii) Take sodium citrate solution (2.94%) or normal saline (0.9%) which is used to dilute semen in the special colorimeteric test tube. Wipe clean with tissue paper and fix into the slot of the colorimeter and switch it on. If needed, adjust the knob and set the needle to show 100 per cent light transmittance.

iii) Take 0.1 ml of neat semen and mix with 9.9 ml of sodium citrate solution or normal saline in a test tube, avoiding air bubbles. From this take aliquot sample into special colorimetric test tube and insert into the slot. Switch on the instrument and note down the light transmittance percentage for the samples.

iv) Find out the concentration of the sperm for the same sample by using a haemocytometer.

v) Repeat with several samples differing in concentration, within the normal range.

vi) Mark the reading in a graph sheet till a straight line is obtained (sperm concentration reckoned by haemocytometer is plotted on X-axis and the light transmittance percentage on Y-axis). Usually 10 to 15 readings within the normal range of concentration will be enough. The sperm concentration of any sample can now be read from light transmittance percentage by referring to the calibration chart.

It is advisable to connect the photoelectric colorimeter to an appropriate voltage stabiliser to avoid errors due to power fluctuations. Periodically the calibration should be checked for its accuracy. For routine dilution of ram semen, visual appraisal of the consistency and deciding the dilution ratio is the most convenient and practical one.

Live and Dead Count

Nigrosin-eosin stain mixture is normally used (Appendix 1). This procedure consists of mixing a drop of semen (immediately after collection) with 10 drops of stain mixture in a test tube, incubating at 30°C for 3 minutes and then drawing smears. Examination of smear and estimation of dead sperm should be done that day itself to avoid the spread of stain to the unstained spermatozoa. If the slides are not examined that day, then they should be mounted in DPX mountant with cover slips and kept in a desiccator until evaluation. A minimum count of 100 spermatozoa in two slides per ejaculate is recommended. Though 200 spermatozoa are normally suggested for examination, practically it is not feasible. Sampling errors are bound to occur due to ejaculate variation, between batches of stain, smear preparation and counting of dead sperm.

The stain mixture is normally stored at 5° for longer periods. A good semen sample should not contain more than 20 per cent dead spermatozoa.

Estimation of Abnormal spermatozoa

Morphological examination of spermatozoa is a detailed test of semen quality. Samples with a high proportion of abnormal spermatozoa can be expected to result in poor fertility. Smears prepared for live and dead count are also used for recording the abnormalities of spermatozoa. Otherwise, Rose Bengal stain is known to give better clarity of abnormalities examined (Appendix 1). The simplest and most practical way to classify abnormalities. is to group them as head, midpiece and tail abnormalities. Abnormalities of the head are considered more serious than those of the tail of spermatozoa. Semen samples containing more than 15 per cent abnormalities are not suited for AI work.

Generally, less native and crossbred rams are rejected from AI Programmes based on quality evaluation. Exotic rams maintained in hotter regions of the country may have to be temporarily withdrawn from breeding during summer season due to deterioration of semen quality.

□□□

16

Dilution, Storage and Freezing of Semen

Diluents

A number of diluents have been tried for storing ram semen as liquid and frozen semen. The proven and most promising diluents and their preparation are given below:

Diluents used for storage as liquid semen

a) Whole milk diluent

Cow milk is easily available, does not require accurate weighing of chemicals.and adjustment of pH. Cow milk is directly obtained in a clean beaker after discarding the first few strips. About 30 ml of cow milk is taken in a test tube and covered with aluminium foil. It should be ensured that either water or water vapour does not enter the milk. A water bath is switched on and when the temperature reaches 95°C the tube containing cow milk is immersed inside the water bath upto the level of the milk. It is kept at 95°C for ten minutes to inactivate the spermicidal factor(s) present in cow milk. Incidentally, boiling also reduces the microbial load of milk.

The milk is cooled down to room temperature and placed overnight in the freezing chamber of the refrigerator. The tube is taken out next day from the refrigerator and the milk is allowed to reach room temperature (30° C). It is then filtered through a thick pad of gauze to make the milk free from large fat globules and cream that had formed. Penicillin (1000 IU/ml) and streptomycin (1 mg/ml) may be added and used for diluting immediately at 30°C or store the antibiotic added diluent in the refrigerator. Such antibiotic added diluents can be stored for 3 or 4 days and a fresh batch can be prepared when needed.

One of the disadvantages of milk diluent is that it is difficult to assess the motility of spermatozoa under the microscope. It requires immediate dilution and use within 12 hours.

b) Sodium citrate-glucose-yolk diluent

Trisodium citrate dihydrate	:	2.37 g
Glucose	:	0.80 g
Egg yolk	:	20 ml
Double glass distilled water to	:	100 ml
Penicillin (IU)	:	100,000
Streptomycin (mg)	:	100

c) Tris-citric acid-fructose-yolk diluent

Tris (hydroxymethyl) aminomethane (0.3 M)	:	3.634 g
Citric acid monohydrate	:	1.99 g
Fructose	:	0.500 g
Egg yolk	:	14 ml
Double glass distilled water added to	:	100 ml
Penicillin (IU)	:	100,000
Streptomycin (mg)	:	100

Source: Evans and Maxwell (1987)

Preparation of the diluents (b and c)

The chemicals should be weighed accurately and transferred to 100 ml capacity measuring cylinder. To this, about 70 ml of double glass distilled water is added and the chemicals are dissolved well. Egg yolk is added and gently mixed with a sterile glass rod. Final volume is made up by adding double distilled water. Penicillin (1000 IU/ml) and streptomycin (1 mg/ml) may be added and the whole diluent should be mixed gently and thoroughly. It should then be transferred to a 100 ml sterile conical flask and covered with aluminium foil. If the diluent is not used immediately, it should be. stored in the refrigerator, but not more than overnight storage. Everyday fresh batch of diluents should be prepared.

Egg yolk

The eggs used should not be more than one week old. If available, it is better to obtain eggs directly from the farm. Otherwise it should be bought from a reliable dealer. Immediately after purchase, the eggs should be stored in a refrigerator without washing or cleaning in any manner. Just before use, the eggs are cleaned thoroughly with 70 per cent alcohol and 'allowed to dry. The egg is cracked at the narrow end and the albumen is drained off by cutting the shell uniformly round with a curved scissors.

The yolk is gently transferred to a circular clean filter peper and the left-over albumen and that sticking on the yolk is absorbed by gently rolling it. During transfer and rolling the yolk, care should be taken to see that the yolk membrane is not ruptured. When free of albumen, the membrane should be ruptured and the yolk is transferred to a sterile beaker by slightly folding the filter paper. The membrane should be retained in the filter paper itself. If yolk is obtained from more than one egg it should be mixed well and then added to the buffer.

Diluents used for Frozen Semen Storage

Both pellet and straw methods of freezing are in vogue. Pelleting is popular in USSR and Australia and straws are generally used in Europe. One step or two-step dilution (popular in France) is adopted depending on the diluent, glycerol level and freezing method. From practical stand-point, one-step dilution and straw-freezing are the most convenient, since they involve less handling of spermatozoa and facilitate accurate measurement of insemination dose, efficient storage and transport of frozen semen.

French medium (0.5 ml) straws are ideal for frozen storage and insemination. The recommended diluents for freezing in straws are:

a) Tris (hydroxyrnethyl) aminomethane : 3.634 g

Citric acid monohydrate : 1.990 g

Glucose : 0.500 g

Egg yolk : 15 ml

Glycerol : 5 ml

Penicillin (lU) : 100,000

Streptomycin (mg)	:	100
Double glass distilled water to	:	100 ml

b) The diluent used by us for freezing and insemination in our laboratory is as follows:

Tris buffer	:	
Tris (hydroymethyl) aminomethane	:	3.48 g
Citric acid monohydrate	:	1.700 g
Fructose	:	1.250 g
Double glass distilled water	:	85 ml
Penicillin (IU)	:	1000/ ml
Streptomycin (mg)	:	1/ ml
pH	:	6.75

Four parts (80 ml) of tris buffer is thoroughly mixed with 1 part (20 ml) of egg yolk. Five ml of the diluent is pipetted out and discarded. Glycerol (5 ml) is added to the measuring cylinder making the volume to 100 ml and mixed well.

Method of Dilution

Dilution serves the twin purposes of extending the semen volume and prolonging the lifespan of spermatozoa. About 15 minutes before collection, freshly prepared diluent is kept in a water bath at 30°C. The suitable containers are 30 ml/10 ml round bottom screw cap vials. The level of the water in the bath should be slightly above that of the diluent. Dilution of semen should be done soon after collection and preliminary evaluation, It is advisable to dilute the semen for AI work within 5 minutes after collection. Known quantity of semen is pipetted out and transferred to a clean sterile test tube in the water bath. Then appropriate quantity of the diluent is added to the semen and mixed gently by aspirating through the pipette and then allowing the diluted semen to flow down on gravity. The dilution ratio should never exceed 1:4 whether used as liquid semen or frozen semen. Generally ram semen used for AI is not diluted based on the actual count of spermatozoa. Consistency of the semen is a simple guide for routine use in A.I. The following dilution ratios are suggested for practical use; but estimation of concentration of spermatozoa will be an accurate guide. In addition, the semen used for dilution should have a mass activity score of 5 or 4.

Consistency of semen	Dilution ratio		
	(Semen	:	Diluent)
Very thick creamy	1	:	4
Thick creamy	1	:	3
Creamy	1	:	2
Thick milky (young rams)	1	:	1

For frozen semen the same dilution ratios can be adopted for one-step dilution. If two-step dilution is followed, out of the total quantity of diluent calculated, initial dilution is made with half the quantity of non-glycerolated diluent at 30ºC. The other half (glycerolated diluent containing double the final concentration of glycerol) can be added when the diluted semen reaches 5°C.

The diluent and semen should be at 30°C to avoid thermal shock. Immediately after dilution a very thin drop of semen is examined under the high power for estimating the percentage of progressively motile spermatozoa. Good semen samples will have more than 70 to 80 per cent of the spermatozoa progressively motile.

Cooling of Liquid Semen for Short-Term Storage

Ram spermatozoa are very much susceptible to cold shock and hence slow cooling is essential. The diluted semen should be brought to 5°C in 3 to 4 hours. The standard practice is to keep 5 ml vials (filled upto the top without air space) in a 100 ml beaker with water (30°C) and place it in the lower chambers of the refrigerator for about 1 hour. Then the beaker with semen vial may be kept in the upper chambers of the refrigerator (but should not be kept in freezing chamber) till use. The amount of water in the beaker may be adjusted in such a way that the diluted semen reaches 5°C in 31/2 to 4 hours. Semen thus stored has to be used within 24 hours, but it is preferable to use within 12 hours. The general practice is to collect semen daily in the breeding season and use the semen soon after dilution and a portion of the diluted semen preserved for insemination in the evening.

Though sperm stored at 5°C maintain good motility for 2 or 3 days, the fertility results would be disappointing.

Cooling of Liquid Semen for Transport

Pre-cooling of diluted semen is not essential if the semen is transported and used for insemination. During transit it is advantageous to use small tubes (2 to 3 ml) with no or little air space at the top. Semen shippers of 1 or 2 pint capacity are ideal for transport. The diluted semen in vials should be wrapped in non-absorbent cotton individually and placed in a beaker (100 ml/50 ml). The beaker can be covered by a polythene cover and secured to make it water tight. The shipper can be filled with sufficient quantity of crushed ice. Direct contact of the breaker with ice can be avoided by keeping waste rubber liners between ice and beaker. Then the lid of the shipper can be closed and the semen is ready for transport. Slow cooling takes place during transit and the semen can be transported safely for 2 to 3 hours without much loss in fertility. The shipper should always be kept in upright position and jerks and jolts should be avoided during transport.

Cooling of Diluted Semen for Freezing

After dilution (at 30° C.) with diluent containing glycerol (one-step dilution), the vials containing diluted semen should be placed in a beaker (100 ml capacity) with water (30°C). The beaker is then placed in a plastic tray (bread box) with water at the same temperature. The plastic tray is placed in the lower chamber of the refrigerator. After about 30 minutes, the tray can be placed in the upper chamber of the refrigerator. If cold handling cabinet is available then the tray can be placed in it immediately after dilution. Whatever be the cooling method, along with diluted semen, polyvinyl alcohol powder (PVA powder), cotton wool, freezing rack and paper towel are also kept so that they can be pre-cooled.

About 1½ hours after placing in cooling equipment, the temperature of the water around the beaker is checked with an alcohol thermometer. By now the temperature would be around 10°C. By practice, the amount of water can be adjusted to get the required rate of cooling.

Crushed ice can be added carefully in small quantities to the water in the tray so that the temperature is brought down to 4 or 5°C. At the end of 2 hours the temperature of the water in the beaker reaches 4 or 5°C which should be checked. Under tropical climate it takes longer time to reach 5°C in the refrigerator. Addition of ice and checking with a thermometer ensures cooling to 5°C. The diluted semen should be at this temperature at least for one hour which is done by adding crushed ice periodically. Then the semen is filled in the French medium (0.5 ml) straws (IMV, France) using a filling comb attached to a vacuum pump. After fifing the straws, it is important to leave a small air space at the open end of the straw. Then the open end is sealed with PVA powder placed in a petri dish. After wiping the excess powder with pre-cooled cotton wool, the straws are put in the plastic tray with water at 4°C or 5°C and allowed to seal the open end for 30 minutes. The identification of the rams and other treatments are done using different colours of straws and sealing powder.

The straws are taken out and dried in pre-cooled towels and kept in freezing racks at 5°C for another 30 minutes. Cooling, filling of semen in straws and drying of straws and keeping it in freezing racks should be carried out inside the refrigerator/cold handling cabinet. Care should be taken to see that the cold chain is not broken and increase in temperature should always be kept under check. Filling in straws after cooling to 5°C and keeping it at that temperature for one hour helps to examine the motility of the spermatozoa before filling. Samples with less than 60 per cent motility can be discarded and thereby avoiding wastage of straws. After keeping the straws in the freezing racks for 30 minutes in the upper chamber of refrigerator freezing process can be started.

The most convenient container for freezing is a thermocole box of 45 x 25 x 30 cm dimension. Liquid nitrogen is poured to 3 inches depth and closed air tight with a thick glass plate for two minutes for vapour pressure to build up and stabilise. The freezing rack with straws and a goblet are placed in the thermocole box and closed for about 10 minutes. The straws should be placed 4.0 to 4.5 cm above the level of the liquid nitrogen. After 10 minutes the frozen straws are quickly collected in the pre-cooled goblet and plunged into the liquid nitrogen in the box and then the goblet is transferred to a liquid nitrogen container swiftly, for storage.

Alternatively, the diluted semen can be filled in the straws (30° C) and sealed with PVA powder. Leaving of small air space is essential to prevent cracking of straws during freezing. The straws are kept in a plastic tray and allowed to cool to 5°C in 2 hours in the refrigerator.

The straws are kept at 5°C for one hour in the plastic tray with water. Crushed ice can be added in small quantities to maintain the temperature. The straws can be dried with paper towels and then kept at 5°C in the freezing rack for half an hour. The process of freezing and storing is similar to the method described earlier.

Thawing of Straws

The frozen straws kept in the containers can be taken out, thawed and evaluated or used for insemination as follows:

The neck plug is removed and straw picking forceps is precooled for about 30 seconds. The canister (properly labelled) is disengaged from the slot and rotated by 180°. It is lifted upto the lower half of the neck. The required straw (only one at a time) is picked within 10 to 15 seconds. If it takes more time, the canister can be lowered and kept for 2 minutes and then lifted again. Immediately after picking the required straw the canister is lowered and the straw is shaken vigourously once or twice and plunged into water at 37° C. The straw is allowed to thaw for one minute.

Evaluation of Frozen Semen

Percentage of progressively motile spermatozoa

Examination of motility of spermatozoa is the simplest test for assessing the quality of frozen-thawed semen. The straw is held in a clean dry test tube and both ends of the straw are cut and frozen-thawed semen is transferred. A small drop is placed on a grease-free clean warm slide and the percentage of progressively motile spermotozoa (which usually varies between 0 and 60 per cent) is estimated. If the spermatozoa are too crowded, the sample may suitably be diluted with spare diluent at 37°C and examined under the high power after placing a cover slip. When motility is low it is advisable to repeat the examination with some more samples from the same straw. If necessary, one more straw from the same ejaculate can be taken out and examined. Semen samples with 40 per cent or higher post-thaw motility are retained for insemination with proper labelling and those with less motility are discarded. Batches with 30 to 40 per cent post-thaw motility may be rechecked to avoid wastage of germ plasm. Even with careful and controlled freezing procedures the rejection rate of frozen semen may be as high as 50 per cent .

Semen of some rams is found to freeze better and the rejection rates are low.

Incubation at 37°C

The frozen-thawed semen can be incubated at 37°C for 1 to 3 hours. This in vitro test is useful as it simulates the activity of spermatozoa under natural conditions. Sample straws from individual ejaculates of ram semen (frozen-thawed) can be incubated for 3 hours. Straws from ejaculates having 30 per cent or more motility after incubation can be used for insemination. However, this test cannot be put to routine use.

Acrosomal damage

Giemsa staining can be used to assess the extent of acrosomal damage as a result of freezing and thawing. Stained slides are examined under oil immersion objective. A minimum of 100 spermatozoa may have to be examined for each sample. The abnormalities include swollen, separating and entirely lost acrosomes. The damage to acrosome does not necessarily impair motility of spermatozoa. As the acrosomal enzymes are involved in oocyte penetration, damage of the acrosome may adversely affect the fertilising capacity of the spermatozoa. Generally not more than 70 per cent of the thawed spermatozoa should have damaged acrosome. Examination of damaged acrosome is laborious and hence the technique is of limited practical value.

❑❑❑

17

Insemination of Ewes

Preparation of Females for Breeding

Highest conception rates are generally obtained in the natural breeding season. The ewes ear-marked for breeding (natural or artificial) must be given special attention 3 or 4 weeks before the onset of breeding season. Vaccination, drenching and shearing must be completed before this period. Nutritional status may be raised by feeding 150 to 200 grams of concentrate mixture 15 days before the start of the breeding season. Weaning of lambs must be completed before including the ewes to AI programme as lactating ewes are known to give lower conception rates.

Heat Detection

Though the sheep in temperate regions are seasonal breeders, indigenous breeds of sheep are known to come in oestrus throughout the year. Sheep are short-day breeders and variation in day length is not pronounced in the tropics because of the nearness to the equator. Lowered atmospheric temperature and availability of fodder during breeding are conducive for higher conception rate.

Heat symptoms are not overt in ewes and hence use of teaser rams is the only way for detection of oestrus. Aproned rams are generally used for heat detection. For efficient heat detection one ram for every 30 or 40 ewes is required and the flock size must not exceed 250 ewes. It is advisable to detect ewes in oestrus twice daily preferably before 7 A.M. and after 5 P.M. Ewes in oestrus seek out the rams and move around them. When mounted they stand still. Such ewes are drafted separately in a holding pen and marked for identification. The average length of the oestrous cycle in ewes is 17 days varying between 13 and 19 days. In the normal breeding season about 5 per cent of the ewes will be detected in oestrus daily during the first cycle.

The average duration of oestrus is 24 hours which usually varies from 12 to 36 hours. One or two semen collections must be made every week in the teaser rams to maintain libido.

Time of Insemination

Usually ovulation takes place 25 to 30 hours after the onset of oestrus. Therefore it is advisable to inseminate ewes 10 to 12 hours after the onset of oestrus. The recommended practice is to inseminate the ewes detected in oestrus in the morning that day evening and those ewes detected in the evening next day morning. If double insemination is performed, first insemination may be done immediately after heat detection and the second one at 10 to 12 hours after the first insemination. The convenient practical schedule will be single insemination during first cycle and double insemination (or natural service) for the second and third cycles. When single insemination is practised, semen collected in the morning can be: diluted and used for inseminating those; ewes detected in oestrus previous day evening. A portion of the diluted semen from each, ram can be stored in the refrigerator for about 8 hours and used for inseminating those ewes detected in oestrus that day morning.

Insemination

The ewes allotted for insemination must be held in a pen without distrurbing much during insemination. The hind quarters of the ewe is lifted by an assistant standing over and facing opposite to the ewe. The ewe is controlled by folding the hind legs at the hock joint. The vulva should be facing the sun to provide adquate light. The external genitalia is wiped clean with moist cotton' wool or dry' tissue paper. A thick cylindrical glass vaginal speculum (15 cm x 1.5/1.75 cm) is lubricated outside with liquid paraffin. Narrower speculum is used for maiden ewes. The speculum is gently introduced into the 'vaginal canal by parting the lips of the vulva and then gently rotated downwards. In' ewes, the cervix - is not always. located at the centre and some practice is required to' locate the" cervix. By' moving the speculum sideways, downwards or towards the centre, the, cervix can be located. Cervix is a hard structure with mucosal folds and slightly hyperaemic. If excess mucus is found, it can be drained, by lowering the hind quarters with speculâm in position.

If neat semen or diluted' semen (immediately after dilution/short-term stored) is used for insemination, the following procedure is adopted, A 0.1 or 0.2 ml graduated pipette is fitted air tight to a rubber bulb. Tip of the pipette is introduced into the semen vial after slightly pressing the rubber bulb with the thumb. Semen is sucked up to' the required level by slightly releasing the pressure on the bulb. Then the semen in the pipette is held without moving up or down by controlling the pressure on the bulb with the thumb. After locating the cervix, the pipette is introduced through the speculum. The tip of the pipette is introduced into the first fold of cervical canal and bulb is pressed to expel the semen. Before expelling the semen, the speculum should be withdrawn slightly to avoid the back flow of semen into the vagina. Due to the tortuous, and narrow cervical canal it is difficult to introduce the pipette beyond one or two cervical folds. Hence, it is almost impossible to deposit the semen in the midcervix or uterus. The speculum and pipette are then withdrawn and the inseminated ewe is released into a holding pen.

Usually, only 0.1 or 0.2 ml is used for cervical insemination. Separate speculum has to be used for each ewe. Though it is advisable to use a separate pipette for each ewe, the routine practice is to use the same pipette for the ejaculate from one ram. However, if the pipette gets contaminated after one or two inseminations it should be changed. A separate assistant is required to record the sire number, ewe, number, the stage of oestrus and volume of the inseminate. Unnecessary conversation during insemination will result in errors while recording and hence avoided. During insemination the ewes should be handled, gently. Chasing the ewes, shouting and rough handling should be absolutely avoided as these practices will reduce conception rate by impairing transport of spermatozoa in the reproductive tract.

Frozen semen insemination involves thawing of straws for 1 minute at 37°C, wiping the straws dry and loading them into the medium straw gun. The procedure for taking straws has been described earlier. The insemination gun is 31.5 cm long and resembles the one used for cows except the length. The plunger is withdrawn to a sufficient length (15 cm) and the straw should be loaded with laboratory seal at the tip. The tip is cut for about 1 cm at right angle. Cutting obliquely will result in the leakage of semen. A suitable sheath (IMV, France) is slipped on and secured tightly using the ring at the bottom. Now the gun is ready for insemination. (In the initial stages of use of frozen semen, a minute drop of semen can be expressed from the loaded AI gun after discarding the first drop and examined under the high power to check the motility). Using a glass speculum and locating the cervix, the frozen semen can be discharged in the first fold of the cervix by pressing the plunger. It should be ensured that the semen is completely expelled. Then the sheath and straw are discarded.

Dose of Semen and Number of Spermatozoa

Normally ram semen is diluted 1:1 to 1:4 depending on the consistency or concentration of semen. Liquid semen is inseminated at the rate of 0.1 ml/0.2 ml per insemination. Each dose of inseminate (freshly diluted) must contain a minimum of 100 million motile spermatozoa. For short-term stored semen 0.15 to 0.20 ml can be used so that a minimum of 150 million motile spermatoza are deposited. If short-term stored semen is used the sample should have at least 70 per cent of spermatozoa in a progressively motile state. It is better to use more spermatozoa than the recomended as one will be erring only on the safe side. If less number of ewes are to be inseminated, then the dilution ratios can be restricted to 1:3 or 1:2. For liquid semen insemination, it is not advantageous to use more than 0.3 ml per dose.

Semen is normally frozen in medium straws (0.5 ml) and each straw at the time of filling should contain 450 to 500 million motile spermatozoa (i.e. 900 to 1000 million/ml). After freezing and thawing, the spermatozoa in each straw should have a minimum of 40 per cent post-thaw motility. Thus each dose of frozen semen should have a minimum of 180 to 200 million motile spermatozoa.

Reports are, conflicting on the use of single versus double insemination in a particular heat period. Marginally higher conception rates have been recorded for double insemination, but it is not worth the extra labour involved. Furthermore, where pedigree records are important, semen from the same ram has to be used at the second insemination. This may be practically difficult when the number of ewes involved is large. If double insemination is practised, adequate number of motile spermatozoa per dose should be deposited at each insemination (according to the type of semen used). It must be borne in mind that results are highly variable with frozen semen and sometimes even disappointing.

Inseminated ewes may be marked (in the head, withers or rump) with dilute acriflavin or picric acid solution (The dyes last sufficiently long but do not stain the wool permanently). For the purpose of heat detection, the inseminated ewes need not be re-introduced for 12 days. Then they can be mixed with the general flock for regular heat detection. During the second cycle, the position of the dye mark can be changed to some other region of the body. The rate of return to oestrus among inseminated ewes is a rough guide for the evaluation of AI programme. If ewes bred to a particular ram return in relatively more numbers, then such rams should be withdrawn from the programme and the cause of low conception rate should be thoroughly investigated. First cycle is ideal for testing any new treatment or technique without adversely affecting the flock fertility. Normally the breeding season is for a span of 45 to 50 days spread over three oestrous cycles. Generally, the conception rates will be lower in primiparous ewes than in pluriparous ewes. Pregnancy rates are, also known to be lower for lactating ewes as compared to dry ewes. In addition, a variety of factors can influence the reproductive function of ewes including instrinsic factors such as age and breed, and extrinsic factors such as nutrition, temperature and season.

Pregnancy diagnosis is not normally practised as there is no simple and reliable method. Satisfactory conception rates can be obtained when semen is used immediately after dilution and the lambing rates will vary between 60 and 70 per cent for all the three cycles. For short-term stored semen the lambing rate will be around 50 per cent. When cervical insemination is done, the results with frozen semen are highly variable (25 to 40 per cent) and therefore semen of outstanding sires alone need to be frozen and used. Rams are found to differ in their fertility levels and this is known to be heritable. The extent of genetic control on fertility needs to be worked.

Oestrus Synchronisation

Synchronisation of oestrus helps to avoid the laborious process of heat detection. In this method all animals are made to come to heat on a predetermined date and insemination (single/double) is carried out at particular time after the withdrawal of the exogenous hormone/ analogue. Since all lambings occur within a short duration, care and management of new-born lambs and suckling ewes can be better organised. Off-season lambings can be adjusted in such a way that maximum market price is there and adequate feed resources are available during growing period.

Progesterone impregnated sponges are the most convenient ones for routine use. Each intravaginal sponge is impregnated with progesterone analogue, Flurogestone acetate and cotton string is firmly threaded through the sponge. The sponge is inserted into the vagina with the help of an applicator consisting of a plastic tube and a rod. However, for indigenous sheep, glass speculum and glass rod are convenient to use. The hind quarters of the ewe are lifted and held secure by flexing at the hock. The glass speculum is lubricated and introduced into the vagina gently as there will be difficulty in insertion during non - oestrous periods. The sponge must be pushed deep up to the cervix and then the speculum is withdrawn. During all these operations care must be taken to see that no injury is caused to the vaginal mucous membrane. The thread attached to the sponge is allowed to hang slightly outside the vagina. The treated ewes should be clearly marked for easy identification at the time of withdrawal.

The sponge is allowed to remain in the vagina for 14 days and the loss of sponge during this period normally does not exeed 2 to 3 per cent. The timing of removal of sponges is adjusted in such a way that fixed time insemination can be done, during morning or evening hours of the day. The sponge can be removed while the ewe is held firmly in standing position. The string is pulled gently, but firmly in a downward direction. If the string cuts through the sponge then it can be removed using duck bill speculum and long forceps. It should be ensured that sponges are removed from all the ewes. Then 350 to 500 I U of pregnant mare serum gonodotrophin (PMSG) can be injected intramuscularly. The reconstitution of the drug is done just prior to the injection. The administration of PMSG helps to regulate the ovulation and shedding of more ova.

At the time of sponge removal, there is strong smelling discharge from the vagina and the sponge, due to the long progestational phase. This is normal except when the discharge contains blood or pus. In such cases ewes should be treated with antibiotics and excluded from the insemination schedule. All the discarded sponges should be carefully collected and buried safely to avoid accidental ingestion by ewes. The treated ewes will come to heat 36 to 48 hours after sponge withdrawal and during that time the discharge will become normal and clear. Whether the animals show symptoms of heat or not, all the treated ewes are inseminated twice i.e. 48 hours and 60 hours after removal of sponges. It is advisable to use liquid semen with a dilution ratio of 1:1 and the semen should be used immediately after dilution. At each insemination, a minimum of 200 million motile spermatozoa must be introduced to obtain maximum fertility. Heat detection may be started 12 or 13 days after the second insemination since those which did not conceive will be naturally cycling. During this natural oestrus, ewes can be bred by natural service or AI. In general, there will be difficulty in introducing sponge in maiden ewes and such ewes can be excluded from synchronisation programme.

However, oestrus synchronisation is a costly venture and can be adopted only in institutional flocks particularly for maintaining nucleus exotic germ plasm. In these sheep anoestrus may be encountered even during breeding season and therefore progestogens can be used to induce oestrus.

Handling and Storage of Frozen Semen

Frozen straws stored should always be kept immersed in liquid nitrogen. Whatever be the volume of the container a minimum depth of 14 cm of liquid nitrogen should be ensured all the time. If the straws are stored in two tiers then a minimum depth of 27 to 28 cm liquid nitrogen is required to be maintained.

The level of liquid nitrogen can be checked using a dip stick properly calibrated. The stick is dipped slowly after preliminary cooling in the vapour. It is introduced completely, held for a few seconds, withdrawn and waved slightly in the air. Frost is formed upto the level of liquid nitrogen which can be read directly.

Replenishment of liquid nitrogen can be done once a week or fortnight depending on the evaporation rate. Transfer of straws to other goblets is best done under liquid nitrogen in styrofoam containers. While raising a canister, it should not be lifted so high that the semen is above the frost line in the neck of the liquid nitrogen container. To facilitate easy identification of straws they should be properly labelled and straws of same ram should be packed together. Plastic goblets are preferred over aluminium goblets because of less temperature fluctuations.

Final Remarks

Tropical sheep are known to breed almost throughout the year. In flock mating, the ram remains with the flock all the time and it is reasonably assumed that 3 lamb crops can be obtained every 2 years. Artifical insemination, even with freshly diluted semen cannot ensure more than 70 per cent lambing. Furthermore, heat detection in ewes is a laborious and time consuming process and it is not feasible to carryout all through the year. Lambing rates with frozen semen do not usually exceed 40 per cent and should be used only in experimental flocks.

Recent experiments have demonstrated that significantly higher conception rates could be obtained adopting intrauterine (laparoscopic) insemination, instead of cervical insemination. These suggest if the sperm cells can avoid passing through the cervical canal they can be more fertile. It has also been shown that with intrauterine insemination good fertility can be achieved even with radically less number of spermatozoa. As low as 20 to 40 million motile spermatozoa are sufficient to achieve satisfactory pregnancy rates. In our country, frozen semen from superior exotic sires can be used extensively throughout the country by adopting laparoscopic insemination. Oestrus synchronisation coupled with laparoscopic insemination will go a long way in improving the genetic merit of our sheep, especially in nucleus and institutional flocks.

Artificial insemination in sheep can be resorted to in farmers' holdings only when sires of high proven genetic worth have to be used extensively. It is also useful when sires of exotic breeds are to be used for crossbreeding. However, the overall productivity of crossbreds should be significantly superior to that of indigenous sheep. In sheep AI can be adopted as a tool for rapid genetic improvement and may not be used for the sake of introducing a new technology.

❑❑❑

18

Cleaning and Sterilisation of Artificial Insemination Equipment

Proper cleaning, drying, sterilisation and maintenance in sterile condition till use are very essential for successful conduct of any AI. programme. Freshly purchased items should be cleaned and sterlised before use unless the manufacturer indicates that they are "ready-to-use" items.

Immediately after use, artificial vaginas, pipettes, measuring cylinders, beakers, conical flasks, specula etc. should be soaked in water containing some mild antiseptic. If they are left as such after use and allowed to dry in the open, then it will be very difficult to clean. Pipettes may be completely clogged and one may have to discard such pipettes ultimately.

After a day's AI work is over, all the materials to be cleaned are collected together and soaked in warm water containing adequate concentration of detergents. Liquid soap is not recommended as it will be difficult to wash off completely. After soaking in detergent solution for about 2 hours, each item is scrubbed thoroughly. Artificial vagina (both hose and liner) is scrubbed well with a U-foam rubber brush and then dismantled. Test tube brushes are used for cleaning glassware, except pipettes. They are cleaned properly by aspirating the detergent solution several times with the help of a rubber bulb.

Washing is done with tap water and several changes of water are made to make the liners and glassware completely free from traces of detergents. Pipettes are washed by aspirating tap water four or five times. Then, all the items are rinsed well with distilled water. Liners are dried by hanging them with the help of a clip and A.V. hoses are dried by keeping them in upright or slanting position. Glassware, especially the pipettes, are kept in slanting position after shaking several times. Then they are dried by keeping them in an incubator.

It is occasionally necessary to place glassware in a dichromate cleaning solution. The solution will remove stain or residual matter that has accumulated. Dichromate cleaning solution is made by slowly adding 250 ml of concentrated sulphuric acid to 500 ml of water. This mixture is cooled and 100 g of potassium dichromate added. When the dichromate is completely dissolved, increase the volume to 1 litre. Glassware should be soaked overnight in this solution and rinsed in several changes of tap water and two or three changes of distilled water.

Daily sterilisation of A.V. hose may not be necessary; but they can be sterilised by keeping them in boiling water for about 20 minutes. Liners are sterilised by soaking them in 70 per cent ethyl alcohol or isopropyl alcohol for about 10 to 15 minutes and dried by hanging in - dust-free cabinets. In addition, a fine spray of 70 per cent alcohol can be made on the liner after assembling the A.V. Once the hot water is filled, the traces of alcohol will evaporate.

Glassware are sterilised by dry heat treatment. Open ends of beakers, conical flasks, measuring cylinders, *etc.*, are covered with aluminium foil. Pipettes and glass rods are covered with butter paper or aluminium foil and sterilised at 165°C for one hour. The sterilised glassware are kept in sterile condition until use by storing them in an instrument cabinet.

❑❑❑

19

Recording of Data

Proper recording of data and maintenance of records are essential for evaluating the success of Al programmes. In addition, accurate recording of insemination and lambing data helps to note the pedigree of the sheep in experimental flocks. During lambing season, it is advisable to record the data within 24 hours of birth of lambs. The most important registers to be kept are semen collection, semen evaluation and insemination registers. The proformae for the registers are given in Tables 1 to 3. From the inseminator's point of view, the recommended procedure for calculating lambing percentage is to take into account only those ewes that were available at the time of lambing out of those inseminated. In other words, ewes culled and died, from insemination to lambing have to be excluded. About 5 per cent of ewes are known to exhibit gestational oerstrus and this should be borne in mind while recording pedigree and reckoning lambing percentage.

Lambing **percentage**

Number of ewes inseminated	=	300
Number of ewes actually available at lambing out of those inseminated	=	280
Number of ewes lambing	=	160
Lambing percentage	=	57.1 (160/280)

1. Semen Collection and Utilisation Register

Date	Genetic group	Ram No.	Order of Collection	Volume (ml)	Colour and consistency	Mass activity	Dilution	Dilution rate	Motility after dilution (%)

Dose of inseminate	No. of ewes inseminated Natives crossbreds exotics Total	Remarks

2. Semen Evaluation Register

Date	Ram No.	Volume (ml)	Colour and consistency	Mass activity	Motility (%)	Concentration (10^6 / ml)	Percent dead sperm

Percent abnormal Sperm	Remarks

3. Insemination Register

Details of insemination

S.No. **Ewe No.** ______________________________

I cycle			II cycle			III cycle	
Date	Ram No.	Vol. (ml)	Date	Ram No.	Vol. (ml)	Date	Ram
No.	Vol. (ml)						

Result of insemination (Lambed / stillborn / aborted)	Date of Lambing	Sex and No. of Lamb	Remarks

❑❑❑

20

Appendices

Appendix-1 : Staining Procedures for Semen Evaluation

I) Stains

1. Nigrosin (water soluble)
2. Eosin (Y) (water soluble)
3. Eosin (B) (water soluble)
4. Giemsa stain
5. Rose Bengal stain

II) Preparation of stains and staining procedures

1. Nigrosin-eosin stain (for live and dead count)

a) Nigrosin-eosin (Y) stain

About 11 grams of Nigrosin is taken and finely ground for about 30 minutes. The fine grinding is essential because of the difficulty in dissolving nigrosin. Nigrosin-eosin stain mixture is prepared as follows:

Nigrosin (water soluble)	:	10.00 g
Eosin (Y) (water soluble)	:	1.67 g
Trisodium citrate dihydrate	:	2.9 g
Distilled water to	:	100 ml

The stain mixture is prepared by dissolving all the items in water in a round bottommed flask (250 ml) and boiling in a water bath for about 30 minutes. After cooling the volume should be made upto 100 ml and filtered.

Staining procedure: About 10-15 drops of stain mixture is kept in a water bath at 30°C. One drop of ram semen is added immediately after collection with the help of a pasteur pipette and incubated for 3 minutes. The test tube is gently shaken after adding the semen drop for proper mixing of semen and stain.

After incubation, one drop of semen-stain mixture is spread on a slide and dried immediately on a warm table. The spreading should be uniform and thin to facilitate accurate estimation. It is advisable to draw several slides from each semen-stain mixture. Examination of slides is done under the oil immersion at a magnification of 1000x. Dead sperm are stained red or pink in the head and partially stained sperm are also counted as "dead". For routine evaluation it is sufficient if 100 spermatozoa are counted at random without choosing fields. Preference should not be given to clear fields and clumps should also be included. If detailed evaluation is needed, it would be better if 200 sperm are counted on two slides. Evaluation should be done that day itself to avoid an upward bias in dead sperm due to the absorption of stain by unstained sperm.

b) Nigrosin-eosin

This stain mixture is prepared by mixing -1 g of eosin (B) and 5 g of nigrosin in 100 ml of 3 per cent trisodium citrate dihydrate solution.

A clean warm (37°C) grease-free slide is taken and a large drop of nigrosin-eosin mixture is placed and a small drop of semen is placed separately on the same slide. Both semen and stain solution should be at the same temperature, say 30°C. Mixing of semen and stain is done with a glass rod having round ends. Immediately several thin smears are prepared, dried and about 200 spermatozoa from two slides are counted.

2. Rose Bengal stain (for abnormal count)

Semen is diluted 1:10 with 3% sodium citrate dihydrate solution. Smears are prepared from the diluted semen on clean and dry glass slides. These smears are dried in air and stained for 15 minutes in Rose Bengal stain. The slides are washed carefully in tap water, dried in air and examined under oil immersion objuctive. Permanent slides may be prepared by mounting in DPX.

Rose Bengal stain is prepared as follows:

Rose Bengal	:	3 g
Commerical formalin	:	1 ml
Distilled water to	:	100 ml

3. Giemsa staining for acrosome integrity

a) Preparation of stock solution of Giemsa stain

Giemsa stain powder	:	3.8 g
Absolute Methanol (AR)	:	375 ml
Glycerol (AR)	:	125 ml

Giemsa stain is ground with methanol in a glass pestle and mortar. Glycerol is added in small quantities and homogenous solution is made. The stock stain mixture must be stored at 37°C for one week. During this period the stock solution is mixed well for a few minutes every day by shaking the bottle.

b) Preparation of formal saline buffer

Formalin (AR)	:	125 ml
Sodium chloride (AR)	:	10 g
Sodium bicarbonate (AR)	:	0.5 g
Distilled water to	:	1000 ml

C. Preparation of Sorensen's phosphate buffer

To prepare M/15 Na_2HPO_4 solution dissolve 9.5g anhydrous Na_2HPO_4 or 11.9g of $Na_2HPO_4H_2O$ in 1 litre of distilled water. To make M/15 KH_2PO_4 dissolve 9.08 g of KH_2PO_4 in 1 litre of distilled water. Store separately in glass stoppered bottles.

To prepare buffered water for the Giemsa stain, mix the following amounts of solution (in ml) every time afresh.

	pH 6.8	pH 7.0	pH 7.2
M/15 Na_2HPO_4	50.0	61.1	72.0
M/15 KH_2PO_4	50.0	38.9	28.0
Distilled water	900.0	900.0	900.0

d) Preparation of buffered Giemsa solution:

For staining fixed smears of spermatozoa, 3.0 ml of Giemsa stock solution is diluted with Sorensen's M/15 phosphate buffer, (pH 7.0) 2.0 ml and distilled water (35 ml)

Preparation of smear and staining

A drop of diluted semen is smeared on a pre-warmed slide and dried in a current of warm air. It is advisable to prepare 3 or 4 slides for each treatment in experiments. The smears are fixed in buffered formal saline for 15 minutes and then washed in running tap water for 15 to 20 minutes. The smears are dried and immersed in the buffered Giemsa solution for 6 to 8 hrs. The smears are rinsed in distilled water and air dired. Permanent mounts of the slides are prepared by covering with rectangular cover slips and using DPX mountant. Slides are examined at a magnification of 1000x and a minimum of 100 spermatozoa may be examined. Acrosome of a spermatozoa is considered to be normal when the stain is clearly and evenly distributed over the spermatozoa head anterior to the equatorial segment. The acrosome morphology is classsified as intact, damaged and lost acrosomes. Acceptable level in frozen-thawed semen is not more than 70 per cent of damaged and lost acrosomes.

Appendix-2 : List of Chemicals (AR/GR GRADE)

Name of the chemical	Empirical formula	Molecular Weight
1. Trisodium citrate dehydrate	$Na_3C_6H_5O7_2.H_2O$	294.10
2. Citric acid monohydrate	$C_6H_8O_7.H_2O$	210.14
3. Glycerol	$C_3H_5(OH)_3$	92.09
4. D-Fructose	$C_6H_{12}O_6$	180.16
5. D-Glucose	$C_6H_{12}O_6$	180.16
6. Tris (hydroxymethyl) aminomethane	$NH_2C(CH_2OH)_3$	121.14
7. Sodium chloride	NaCl	58.44
8. Potassium dihydrogen orthophosphate	Na_2HPO_4	141.96
9. Disodium hydrogen orthophosphate	Na_2HPO_4	141.96
10. Lactose (lactose monohydrate)	$C_12H_{22}O_{11}.H_2O$	360.32

Appendix-3 : Equipment, Glassware and Accessories Required for AI in Sheep

General Purpose Equipment		No
1. Analytical balance	:	1
2. Hot air oven	:	1
3. Refrigerator 165/286 L	:	1
4. Bacteriological incubator	:	1
5. Light microscope with imported oil immersion objective	:	2
6. Bouble glass distillation apparatus	:	1
7. Deioniser	:	1
8. pH meter	:	1
9. Autoclave	:	1
Collection Equipment		
1. Service crate for sheep	:	2
2. Stove/Kettle	:	2
3. A.V. hose (20 cm x 5 cm)	:	10
4. Liners 30 cm	:	30
5. Collection cups	:	30
6. Warm stage for examination of semen	:	1
Dilution and Cooling		
1. Serological water bath	:	1
2. Cold handling cabinet	:	1
3. Bread box to keep semen vials	:	10
4. Semen shipper (1 pint/2 pints)	:	2
Freezing and Storage		
1. Freezing racks S.S	:	4
2. Thermocole box	:	2
3. Liquid nitrogen containers 3.9,10, & 35 litres capacity	:	1 each
4. Straw picking forceps	:	2 to 4
5. Goblet lifting forceps	:	2
Insemination		
1. Insemination guns (mini/medium)	:	6
2. Glass speculum		

15 cm x 1.50 cm	:	30
15 cm x 1.75 cm	:	20

Glassware

1. a) Pipettes (serological) 1 ml, 2 ml and 5 ml	:	10 each
b) Pipettes (serological) 0.1 and 0.2 ml	:	10 each
2. Glass vials (round bottommed) 5 ml	:	20 each
3. Glass vials 30 ml	:	10
4. Measuring cylinders 25, 50 and 100 ml	:	6 each
5. Beakers 50, 100 and 250 ml	:	6 each
6. Conical flasks 25, 50 and 100 ml	:	6 each
7. Microscopic slides (Blue Star)	:	20 boxes
8. Cover slips (round/square 19 mm) (Blue star)	:	30 boxes
9. Pasteur pipettes	:	20
10. Capillary tubes	:	20 boxes
11. Straws (mini/medium)	:	2000
12. Sheaths (for the above)		
13. Test tubes	:	30
14. Pestle and mortar	:	2

* Borosil glassware are preferred

Accessories

1. Tissue paper
2. Non-absorbent cotton
3. Rubber bulb
4. U-foam rollers
5. Air blower for A.V.
6. A.V. Cleaning brush
7. Brush for cleaning test tube
8. Detergent powder

Appendix-4 : List of firms supplying A.I. and frozen semen equipment for sheep

FOREIGN

Instruments Medicine (IMV)

B.P. 76
10, rue Cle'menceau
61300 L'Aigle
France

INDIAN

A.I. equipment

Ocean Surgicals

Bharwadia Bhawan,
M.I. Road,
Jaipur - 302 001
Rajasthan.

International Traders,

Sharma Buildings,
M.I. Road,
Jaipur - 302 001
Rajasthan.

Ocean Surgical Company

51/2, Desh Bahdhu Gupta Road,
Karol Bagh,
New Delhi - 110 005.

Jayanth Brothers,

425-A, Kilpauk Garden Road,
Chennai- 600 010.

Rajasundary Industries,

Unit No: 12, SIDCO Industrial Estate,
Theni - 626 531.
Madurai (Dt.)
Tamil Nadu.

Shakti Enterprises,

87/B-i, East Azad Nagar,
Delhi - 110 051.

Saarnash Udyog,
A-6 17, Krishna Nagar,
Delhi - 110 055.

Daaps Intraco P. Ltd.,
D- 117, Okhla Industrial Estate, Phase-I, New Delhi - 110 020.

Insemination and Dairy Equipments,
F-4, DSIDC, Industrial Complex,
Rohtak Road,
Delhi - 110 041.

Liquid Nitrogen Containers
IBP **Co., Ltd.,**
Engineering Division,
Sewn (East),
Bombay - 400 015.

Daaps Breeding Products,
1 7-E, Community Centre,
Basant Lok,
New Delhi - 110 057.

Bharat Heavy Plate and Vessels Ltd.,
Visakapatnam - 530 012.
Andhra Pradesh.

Jubilee Medical Engineering Co.,
Vajapeyam Gardens,
7th Cross,
Bangalore - 560 050.

□□□